SuperFoodsRx
for Pregnancy

SuperFoodsRx for Pregnancy

The Right Choices for a Healthy, Smart, Super Baby

STEVEN PRATT, M.D.

WILEY

Cover Design: © HATCHBEAUTY
Cover Photograph: © Stephen Coburn/Shutterstock

Published by John Wiley & Sons, Inc., Hoboken, New Jersey
Published simultaneously in Canada

The information contained in this book is not intended to serve as a replacement for professional medical advice. Any use of the information in this book is at the reader's discretion. The author and the publisher specifically disclaim any and all liability arising directly or indirectly from the use or application of any information contained in this book. A health care professional should be consulted regarding your specific situation.

For general information about our other products and services, please contact our Customer Care Department within the United States at (800) 762-2974, outside the United States at (317) 572-3993 or fax (317) 572-4002.

Wiley also publishes its books in a variety of electronic formats and by print-on-demand. Some content that appears in standard print versions of this book may not be available in other formats. For more information about Wiley products, visit us at www.wiley.com.

ISBN 978-1-118-12954-8 (paper); ISBN 978-1-118-22561-5 (ebk);
ISBN 978-1-118-23836-3 (ebk); ISBN 978-1-118-26303-7 (ebk)

Printed in the United States of America

10 9 8 7 6 5 4 3 2 1

To all those parents—past, present, and future—who work tirelessly to provide the very best for their families, and to the late Dr. James Joseph, whose scientific publications, strong faith in God, and wonderful, cheerful friendship will always be sources of inspiration to those of us who were blessed by his presence

Please register with the SuperFoods team at http://www.superfoodsrx .com/pregnancybook. We will be posting updates, adding tips and recipes, taking questions, and more.

Contents

Acknowledgments

My family always plays a special, and often—at least at the time—underappreciated role in my ability to write a book while still working full time at my "day job" as a physician. My wonderful wife, Gunilla, always brings her cheerfulness, organizational/computer skills, and loving support to my book projects. My seven kids—Michael, Tyler, Torey, Brian, Jennifer, Grant, and Marlaina—give me a sense of purpose, especially when I'm writing about "superbabies." A particular thanks to Grant, a PhD student in the Evolutionary Biology of Diets and Aging, for his scientific help, and to Torey, who once again supplied me with so many of the scientific (especially environmental) publications that are the backbone of any book on health and wellness.

I'm thankful that Kimberly Baker, the world's best librarian, is still employed by Scripps. What a gift she has for tracking down the answers to my get-the-science-correct questions!

As with my previous four books, my SuperFoodsRx partners, Ray Sphire, David Stern, and Dr. Hugh Greenway, have given me their enthusiastic support and counsel for this project.

Thank you to Dr. Victor Sierpina and his wife, Michelle; Dr. Shakha Gillin; and Dr. Nancy Clementino for their helpful advice and willingness to listen to my questions about this important subject.

Thanks to all my office staff for everything they do for me, with special appreciation to Carol Henry, Maurya Troiano, and Taylor Nimmo.

Many of my patients offer plenty of encouragement when I am in "book mode." I want all of you to know that you are really helping to make all the long hours of research and writing worth the effort!

Throughout my book-writing career I have been fortunate to work with great professionals who can turn scientific jargon into interesting material for health-care professionals as well as the lay public. This book is no exception! Thank you, Judy Kern, for your unsurpassed, no-nonsense professionalism in getting this book to the finish line. Judy, you are a real pro!

Thank you John Wiley & Sons for Tom Miller, Lisa Burstiner, Connie Santisteban, and John Simko.

Thank you to my agent, Andrea Barzvi: you have been great, and I really appreciate your friendship and, of course, the amazing job you do in helping to create a book from what was initially nothing more than "I think there is a worldwide need for this book."

Introduction

You Have More Power Than You Think

Ihave great news for all prospective parents: there's a tremendous amount you can do, even before your child is conceived, that will have a lifelong effect on his or her health and well-being. And the bonus is that whatever you do for your unborn child will also benefit you for the rest of your life.

Just a couple of generations ago the general belief was that no matter what an expectant mother ate, drank, or breathed, her baby would grow and thrive, even if the health of the fetus meant that the mother was less well nourished. In other words, the baby's health in utero would be maintained at the expense of the mother's.

We also believed that the placenta would protect the developing fetus from any and all external assaults—that it was an impermeable barrier, and nothing could pass over, under, around, or through it.

Finally, we thought that once the sperm and the egg met and married, nothing could change the genetic blueprint the unborn child had inherited from Mommy and Daddy.

More recently, however, science has shown that none of these previously held beliefs is entirely true. Fetal origins research and epigenetics, two relatively new fields of scientific study, are continuously providing more and more evidence that a mother's and father's prenatal nutrition and environmental exposures have a continuing impact on their unborn child.

Fetal origins research looks at what the unborn child receives from its environment—that is, the quantity and quality of the nutrition as well as the kinds of hormones and other chemicals circulating in the mother's bloodstream. What we have learned from fetal origins research is that far from being immune to external assaults, the fetus is affected by the chemicals, nutrients, and toxins the mother eats, breathes, and even absorbs through the skin, and whatever is found in the mom's bloodstream is also found in the umbilical cord blood and in the newborn's first stool.

Epigenetics investigates the ways these prenatal factors continue to affect the expression of various genes throughout the life of the child and how they can also be passed down to future generations, even though DNA itself does not change. Although it may take hundreds, if not thousands, of years for genetic changes to occur based on natural selection ("survival of the fittest"), epigenetic changes take place over, above, and beyond (in Greek *epi*) the genetic level.

Although a person's basic genetic code is set at the time of conception, there are also variables that determine how, whether, and when particular genes are turned on, or expressed. What this means is that parents have a profound effect on their children, starting well before the cradle and continuing long after the children leave the nest—all the way to the grave and into future generations.

An example of how this works is the phenomenon known as temperature-dependent gene expression, which can be seen in a particular strain of fruit fly, *Drosophila melanogaster*. It normally has white eyes, but if the temperature surrounding its embryos, which is normally 77 degrees Fahrenheit, is briefly raised to 98.6 degrees Fahrenheit, the flies hatch with red eyes. If these flies are then bred with one another, the subsequent generations will be partly red-eyed even though they were not subjected to the temperature change, and the gene responsible for eye color will remain the same for both the red-eyed and the white-eyed flies.

More than twenty years ago, Dr. David Barker, now considered the father of fetal origins research, began to investigate why the poorest regions of England and Wales also seemed to have the highest rates of coronary heart disease. What he discovered was that there was a positive correlation between low birth weight (usually the result of poor prenatal nutrition) and the risk for developing heart disease later in life.

Subsequently Dr. Tessa Roseboom, along with Barker and others, studied the relationship between prenatal exposure to the Dutch famine of 1944 and 1945 and the onset of adult disease.

In the wake of the German embargo on food transport late in 1944, the urban western region of the Netherlands was left without adequate food for the harsh winter months. As food supplies dwindled, rationing became harsher and harsher, until the official daily rations for the area provided only 400 to 800 calories per person per day.

The researchers identified 2,414 babies born in a university hospital in Amsterdam between November 1, 1943, and February 28, 1947, and compared those who were affected by the famine to those who were not. Although disease rates varied according to the length of time and at what period of gestation the fetus was malnourished, they concluded the following:

Our findings broadly support the hypothesis that chronic diseases originate through adaptations made by the foetus in response to undernutrition [and] suggest that risk factors for CHD [coronary heart disease], such as impaired glucose tolerance, hypercholesterolaemia, raised blood pressure, and obesity, which often co-exist, have their origins in utero, but are programmed at different times. Furthermore, our findings suggest that maternal malnutrition during gestation may permanently affect adult health without affecting the size of the baby at birth.

The Barker Theory website (http://www.thebarkertheory.org) further states that "recent findings have shown that a woman's body composition and diet *at the time of conception and during pregnancy* have important effects on the subsequent health of her offspring" (emphasis added).

Fortunately, most of us in the developed world do not suffer from famines, but that does not mean we are always getting optimal nutrition. In fact, affluence, along with easy access to prepared and processed foods, has given us an unprecedented opportunity to make wrong choices as well as right ones. And women who are or who are planning to become pregnant don't always know what choices to make to assure optimal health for themselves and their baby.

In the wake of Barker's findings, there is now a significant and growing body of scientific evidence to show that how we are nourished in utero and during infancy effectively determines our lifelong risk for a wide range of health issues and noncommunicable diseases, including not only cardiovascular disease, diabetes, cancer, hypertension, and obesity but also bone health, intestinal function, immune system strength, age of menarche, depression, anxiety, substance abuse, learning, behavior, and longevity. We each have a specific, immutable genetic code—our "nature." But how our genes are "expressed" (that is turned on or not) is profoundly affected by our early nutrition and environment—the way we are nurtured.

In 2011, Alan A. Jackson of the University of Southampton in England wrote in the *American Journal of Clinical Nutrition*:

> There is now substantial evidence from epidemiologic studies that the shape and size of an infant at delivery and his or her growth during the first two years of life are predictive of later risk of chronic noncommunicable disease, such as cardiovascular disease, obesity, type 2 diabetes, respiratory disease, osteoporosis, cancer, and mental illness. . . . Normal growth and development are highly structured and progress in a way that is strictly ordered in space and time. Any failure to ensure the provision of a mix of nutrients appropriate for the needs at that particular time risks constraining one or another aspect of this complex process.

In *SuperFoodsRx for Pregnancy*, I'm going to answer all of the questions prospective parents might have about how to create the best, most nourishing and nurturing internal and external environment for their child before, during, and after pregnancy. I'll explain exactly which foods—the SuperFoods—to eat and why; which vitamins, minerals, and other supplements have important effects on the health of the developing fetus; and how to avoid the environmental toxins that could negatively affect the health of both parents and child.

Most of the keys to having superhealthy kids are right there in the supermarket, in your cupboard, on your dinner plate, and in your lifestyle choices. You just need to know how to make the right choices and perhaps some small changes in your diet and daily routine. None of this is difficult, and the information I provide shouldn't create more stress in your life. On the contrary, my goal is to relieve the anxiety created by uncertainty so that you are free to enjoy all the pleasures of pregnancy and parenthood to the fullest.

As I was writing, I couldn't help thinking that, if only our parents and grandparents had been able to read this book, they would have increased our chances of avoiding many, if not most, of the diseases of modern humanity. Still, it's never too late to start making changes. In fact, if you're already pregnant when you start to read this book, you can begin to follow my recommendations in order to significantly increase your own health, the health of your child, and even the health of future generations.

Everything you'll be reading is based on rigorous scientific investigation. Some of the findings have already been so thoroughly investigated that they are now incontrovertible. Some are still in the early stages or have not yet been confirmed in humans. In some cases science has not yet proved how or why particular outcomes occur. But even these cases point toward nutritional and lifestyle changes that could well improve your child's chances of living longer and better.

In no case do I suggest anything that could possibly be detrimental, and it seems to me that if increasing your consumption of a particular food or decreasing your exposure to a particular chemical just *might* prove to be good for you and your child, it's certainly worth incorporating into your diet and lifestyle. Do as much as you can, and don't stress about not being perfect. Nobody's perfect, and, as I've said, the purpose of this book is to decrease your stress level, not to add to it.

PART 1

Before You Get Pregnant

I like to call this part of the book prepregnancy boot camp, but it could just as easily be called prepregnancy *boost* camp, because the nutritional and lifestyle changes you make before you get pregnant will increase your fertility, your chances of having a healthy pregnancy and a healthy baby, and your own chances of living a longer and healthier life.

I'm sure you've heard couples proudly announce, "We're pregnant." That is a euphemism in the sense that it is, of course, technically the woman who is pregnant, but the man also plays a big role. Not only is he equally responsible for conception, but in terms of providing a maximally healthy external environment for his future child, he is—or should be—an equal partner.

The first chapter of this book is all about what both potential moms and potential dads can do to increase their chances of becoming pregnant. The percentage of couples who are finding it difficult to conceive is on the rise. There are undoubtedly multiple reasons for this unfortunate phenomenon, such as the increased tendency to delay starting a family, the prevalence of obesity in adults (with all the attendant health issues), and the number of environmental toxins and pollutants to which we are exposed on a daily basis.

Therefore, in chapter 1 you will find separate sections addressed specifically to women and to men. Moms-to-be need to start maximizing their nutrition by consuming as many health-promoting whole foods as possible. So this is where you'll find my list of the twenty-five SuperFoods and their particular benefits. But you may be surprised to learn that this is also when you should begin to cut down on, or even cut out completely, caffeine and alcohol, because studies have shown that the more caffeine and alcohol women consume, the longer it takes them to become pregnant. Tea, on the other hand, has been shown to boost fertility, and it has many other health benefits as well.

Prepregnancy is also when women should be taking control of their weight and losing extra pounds, if necessary. Women who are overweight or obese have a harder time conceiving and also have more pregnancy complications for both themselves and their babies-to-be. I know that weight is a touchy subject, but more and more research is showing that it has a significant effect on our health—possibly more than any other single health factor—so I'll be talking about it throughout this book.

Weight is also an issue for prospective dads, because studies have shown that excess weight is directly related to having an abnormal sperm count. In addition to weight, oxidative stress (an imbalance in our body where there are not enough antioxidants to neutralize the ever-present free radicals) and free radical damage have been correlated with male infertility or subfecundity. So, guys, as you'll see, eating the same antioxidant-rich SuperFoods I recommend for women will boost your sperm count and motility and protect those little swimmers on their long and dangerous journey to meet up with an egg.

Chapter 2 is all about detoxing your external environment—or, as I call it, going green without going crazy. We're surrounded— bombarded, actually—on a daily basis by all kinds of chemicals, some of which are known to be toxic and others that have not been tested, either individually or in combination. These toxins are in a wide range of household and personal care products as well as in the foods we eat and the water we drink.

All of us, but particularly those planning to have a child, should do whatever they can to limit exposure to these toxins, and in this chapter I'll talk about where the majority of them are found as well as how to avoid them as much as possible.

Then, getting back to the woman preparing her body to carry a baby, in chapter 3, I'll talk about a few tests I believe all moms-to-be should take to assess their nutritional and health status before they become pregnant. Once you know where you stand, you'll know what you need to do to get where you want to be. In each area—blood pressure and blood sugar level, vitamin D level, inflammation, anemia, and the blood levels of various nutrients—I'll provide the parameters for optimal health as well as the steps you can take to improve yours.

We'll also discuss how to get the toxins out of your body before there's a baby in your tummy. Detoxing the body is again related to weight, because most of the pollutants we ingest are stored in our fat cells; thus, as we begin to lose fat, we mobilize the toxins into the bloodstream so they can then be eliminated. In this chapter you'll learn about your phase 1 and phase 2 detoxification systems and the simple changes you can make to get them up to speed.

Since not only the nutrients but also the toxins and bacteria in your system are passed on to your baby in utero, you want to be sure that what he or she is getting from you is as health promoting as possible. You may not have heard the term *microbiome*, but it describes the bacteria, good and bad, that all of us have in our bodies. In this chapter we'll talk about what you need to do to clean up your microbiome for your baby, as well as why you need to take care of your oral health and why, once again, you need to take control of your weight.

Finally, at the conclusion of part one, I'll provide you with lists of specific food sources for each of the vitamins, minerals, and other nutrients we've talked about, along with the quantities found in each food, how much of the food you should eat, and how often you need to be eating it. I'll list my own and/or the government's recommendations for how much of each nutrient you should be getting through diet or supplementation.

So now that you know what to expect, it's time to get started.

1

Fast-Track
Your Fertility

Obviously, the first step in having a superhealthy baby is actually getting pregnant and carrying the baby to term. Statistics indicate that infertility—defined as the failure to conceive after twelve months of unprotected intercourse—affects an estimated 6.2 million U.S. women, with projections that there will be 7.7 million infertile women by 2025.

There is also an increasing body of research on the many modifiable lifestyle choices that can significantly increase fertility in both men and women. Male infertility is indeed the sole cause of a couple's inability to conceive a child in a significant number of cases. The so-called male factor appears to be the sole cause for infertility in at least 20 percent of cases and a contributing factor in 30 to 40 percent of cases. In fact, it is estimated that 6 percent of men are infertile during their reproductive years. So you dads-to-be need to listen up, too!

For Women: Eat Your Way to Pregnancy

If you are a woman who is trying to become pregnant, eating more of the foods that have been shown to increase the rate of conception is a simple way to get on the fast track to parenthood. Studies have shown that eating SuperFoods—the twenty-five categories of food that are low on the glycemic index and that mirror what is now generally referred to as the Mediterranean diet—will help to increase fertility. These SuperFoods are listed later in this chapter.

For example, a small study in the Netherlands of women undergoing fertility treatment found that of the 161 participating couples, the women who were following a diet that most closely resembled the Mediterranean diet were 40 percent more likely to become pregnant than those whose diet was least like the Mediterranean diet.

One reason this diet might contribute to increased fertility is that it generally contains a healthy balance of omega-3 (alpha-linolenic acid and marine omega-3s—that is, EPA, DHA, and others) and omega-6 (linoleic acid) fatty acids. Both omega-3 and omega-6 are essential fatty acids; the body cannot manufacture them and must obtain them from food sources. We'll be talking much more about the many health benefits of omega-3 later in the book. For now, let's look at how and why healthy omega-6 might increase your chances of becoming pregnant.

Most Americans actually consume too much omega-6 and not enough omega-3, and a high percentage of our omega-6 consumption comes from unhealthy sources such as processed foods, cakes, cookies, and other pastries, which are known to promote inflammation, without the adequate consumption of counterbalancing anti-inflammatory omega-3. However, the Mediterranean diet, like the SuperFoods diet, provides optimum *healthy* sources of omega-6 and omega-3, both of which are precursors to substances in the body called prostaglandins, which in turn are involved in regulating the menstrual cycle and initiating ovulation. Up to three times as much omega-6 as omega-3 is the ideal ratio. Since having a normal menstrual cycle is likely to make it easier to become pregnant, eating foods rich in health-promoting sources of these essential fatty acids will promote conception.

SuperFood Sources of Omega-6
- Walnuts
- Corn and corn oil
- Peanuts and peanut oil
- Soybean oil
- Sunflower seeds
- Whole grains
- Ground flaxseed meal
- Chia seeds
- Pumpkin seeds
- Sesame seeds
- Pecans

Get More Vitamin C

Vitamin C is not just in orange juice, although that is certainly a great fruit source. It's also in bell peppers and vegetables like broccoli and Brussels sprouts, and when taken during hormonal stimulation by women undergoing in-vitro fertilization, it has been shown to increase the number of pregnancies achieved. The assumption, therefore, is that it will also improve the pregnancy rate in women who are not in fertility treatment.

So eating foods rich in vitamin C could help to increase your chances of becoming pregnant. And if you're also smoking (which you absolutely shouldn't be, because smoking has a negative effect on fertility), you'll need it even more, since smoking depletes your body of vitamin C and other important nutrients that are essential for a healthy baby and a healthy life. For a list of foods rich in vitamin C, see chapter 4.

Gear Up Your Glutathione

Glutathione and its family of antioxidant enzymes is found inside every cell (what I like to call the cell's primary missile defense system) and works with other antioxidants—such as vitamin C, alpha-lipoic acid, and selenium—to protect DNA from damage, boost the immune system, detoxify the body, and decrease inflammation. High levels of glutathione have also been correlated with a decrease in the time it takes to get pregnant.

SuperFood Sources of Glutathione

- Asparagus
- Avocados
- Black pepper (enhances the liver's production of glutathione)
- Broccoli
- Grapefruit
- Oatmeal
- Oranges
- Peanut butter
- Spinach
- Walnuts
- Watermelon

Most of the glutathione in our cells is manufactured by our bodies. A good way to increase cellular glutathione is to eat more foods containing cysteine, one of only two amino acids that contain sulfur, because the sulfur-containing amino acids provide an important component of glutathione.

SuperFood Sources of Cysteine

- Turkey, skinless breast
- Chicken, skinless breast
- Yogurt, always nonfat and preferably organic
- Eggs, free-range, if possible

- Soy
- Cold-water fish (such as sockeye salmon)
- Whey protein
- Red bell peppers
- Oats
- Garlic
- Onions
- Broccoli
- Brussels sprouts
- Wheat germ

Consuming 10 to 20 grams of one of these sources of cysteine shortly after you get up in the morning will rev up your glutathione production, thus ensuring that your body is being adequately protected throughout the day.

Increase Your Antioxidants

All of the foods listed above are great sources of antioxidants, the naturally occurring chemicals that reduce both oxidative stress, by neutralizing free radicals in the body, and the inflammation that occurs at the cellular level from free radical damage. Although there are no overt symptoms of this inflammation, it is the precursor of many chronic diseases, including arthritis, osteoporosis, cardiovascular disease, stroke, cancer, dry-eye syndrome, age-related macular degeneration, and diabetes. Your body is an incredibly complicated machine, but when it's overstressed it isn't functioning efficiently, and among the many functions affected will be your ability to conceive.

One of the most important antioxidants for trying to conceive may be beta-carotene, because a significant amount of it surrounds and protects the oocyte, or immature egg. So it makes sense to be sure that there are adequate amounts of this particular phytonutrient surrounding your eggs. (For a list of foods rich in beta-carotene, see chapter 7.)

That said, to keep all of the cells in your body running smoothly, you need to eat a wide range of SuperFoods that are rich in all of the antioxidants.

The SuperFoods and What They Do

The following is my list of twenty-five SuperFoods, along with what I call their sidekicks, other foods in the same category that also supply a good amount of the same nutrients but for which fewer studies have been done. See chapter 4 for the quantities of each food to aim for in your diet.

Apples (and Pears, Bananas, and Pineapple)

An apple contains only about 5.7 milligrams of vitamin C, but the antioxidant protection it provides is equivalent to taking approximately 1,500 milligrams of vitamin C in supplement form.

The polyphenol antioxidants found in apples have been shown to protect the body from cardiovascular disease, various cancers, and other medical conditions associated with oxidative stress and inflammation. (*Polyphenols* are one type of the more than eight thousand antioxidant compounds widely dispersed in the plant kingdom.) By altering gene expression, apples can inhibit the enzyme systems known as lipoxygenase and cyclooxygenase, both of which produce inflammatory chemicals called cytokines. A recent epidemiological study has shown that people who consume larger amounts of apple polyphenols can cut their risk for colon cancer (the second leading cause of cancer-related death in the United States) by nearly 50 percent.

At least 10 percent of lung cancer cases occur in people who are not smokers. In two major studies, the Nurses' Health Study and the Health Professionals' Follow-Up Study, fruit and vegetable intake was linked to a 21 percent reduced rate of lung cancer in women, and of the fruits and vegetables evaluated, apples were among those specifically correlated with a decreased rate of lung cancer. In addition, scientists at Cornell University who have done animal research on apples and breast cancer found that the human equivalent of one apple a day reduced the rate of lung tumors in lab rats by 25 percent, and the equivalent of three apples reduced the rate by up to 61 percent.

It's interesting to note that most of the polyphenols in apples are contained in the skin and that apples with different skin colors have different polyphenol contents. So it would be a good idea to eat as many different types of apples as you can. One unique polyphenol in apple skins, phloridizin, mitigates the effects of glycation, a chemical process caused by excess sugar that leads to premature aging, by blocking the transport of glucose from the intestines into the blood stream.

Consumption of apples, particularly of the polyphenols in the skin, has also been shown to have an aspirin-like effect by reducing the stickiness of blood platelets, thus helping to prevent the formation of dangerous blood clots.

Another health-promoting characteristic of apples is their ability to lower LDL (bad) cholesterol and triglycerides, while slightly raising HDL (good) cholesterol, and to reduce the accumulation of visceral (abdominal) fat, which is a major risk factor for cardiovascular disease, diabetes, and cancer. HDL cholesterol contains natural antioxidant molecules known as paraoxonases, and in one rat study, unfiltered apple juice and the accompanying apple polyphenols increased paraoxonase activity by as much as 23 percent.

Numerous studies have correlated the consumption of apples or apple juice with a decreased rate of asthma. A study from the Netherlands followed the diets of 2,000 women and the lung health of 1,253 of their children and found that apples were the only food eaten by the pregnant women that showed a consistent correlation with protection from childhood wheezing and/or asthma.

The children of the women who ate four or more apples per week had a 53 percent lower rate of asthma.

In addition to producing all of the above benefits, apples have been shown to reduce symptoms from seasonal allergies, such as runny nose and sneezing, and there is early suggestive evidence that they can play a role in preventing atopic dermatitis (a type of eczema that often occurs along with other allergic reactions such as hay fever, allergic conjunctivitis, and asthma). Apples also boost immunity, and studies have shown that they can provide protection from several common bacterial pathogens, including staph aureus (commonly known as staph infections), pseudomonas, atypical tuberculosis infections, *Helicobacter pylori* (a common cause of ulcers), and the H1N1 (swine flu) virus. There is at least one animal study showing that apples may even help to prevent osteoporosis and increase bone-mineral density.

For more on how apples can protect you and detoxify your body from environmental pollutants, see chapter 3.

CONSUMER ALERT

Let's ask food companies to make an applesauce that contains the skins. I'm sure it can be done!

Avocados (and Asparagus and Artichokes)

Avocados are dense in calories, but they are also extremely dense in nutrients and fiber, and they contain more folate, potassium, vitamin E, and magnesium than any other fruit. In fact, they contain more magnesium, which is essential for healthy bones and cardio-vascular health, than any of the twenty most commonly eaten fruits. In addition, research has shown that some other nutrients, including the carotenoid antioxidants lycopene, lutein, and beta-carotene, are absorbed more efficiently when eaten with avocados. So by all means have some guacamole, eat some avocado on whole-wheat toast, or include avocado chunks in your salad along with carrots and tomatoes.

Beans (including Pinto, Kidney, Navy, Great Northern, Lima, Garbanzo, and Green Beans; Lentils; and Sugar Snap and Green Peas)

Also called *legumes* because they have a pod with seeds inside, beans are among the best sources of vegetarian protein. One cup of lentils, for example, has about the same amount of protein as two ounces of extra-lean sirloin steak, but the steak has about six times more fat. One of the best things about beans is their ability to help you stabilize your blood sugar level, which, as we'll be discussing throughout this book, is the key not only to weight control but also to reducing your risk of a wide range of serious chronic diseases.

Legumes are low on the glycemic index, which means that they don't cause the blood sugar level to spike; they're also low in calories and inexpensive. In addition to being a good source of vegetarian protein, beans contain high amounts of dietary fiber, prebiotics (the key for health-promoting probiotic bacteria), and polyphenols, as well as other bioactive phytonutrients.

A number of studies have shown an inverse relationship between a legume-based diet and the rates of cardiovascular disease, obesity, type 2 diabetes, and some forms of cancer. The consumption of nonsoy legumes is correlated with small waist circumference, low body weight, decreased systolic (the top number) blood pressure, improved blood glucose level, and a reduced rate of all of the causes of cardiovascular death.

Markers, in medicine, are traits, conditions, and very often blood chemicals that, when present or elevated beyond what has been established as "normal," indicate the presence of or a probable increased predisposition for a condition or disease. Beans are high in magnesium as well as in fiber, and both have been correlated with reduced levels of C-reactive protein and other markers for inflammation.

For all of these reasons, we in the United States would be wise to follow the lead of many traditional diets in other parts of the world and add more beans to our diet.

Blueberries (and Purple or Green Grapes, Cranberries, Boysenberries, Raspberries, Goji Berries, Strawberries, Currants, Blackberries, Cherries, and All Other Varieties of Fresh, Frozen, or Freeze-Dried Berries)

The list of vital nutrients in blueberries is longer than that of virtually any other food. They are heart-healthy, with the ability to raise HDL cholesterol. But perhaps one of their greatest assets is their ability to protect the brain from the degenerative effects of oxidative stress, thereby preventing the development of age-related diseases such as Parkinson's and Alzheimer's.

One study showed that rats given the human equivalent of one cup of blueberries per day for two months had improved balance, coordination, and memory. My late friend Dr. James A. Joseph, the former director of the Human Nutrition Research Center on Aging at Tufts University in Massachusetts, found that blackberries, cranberries, strawberries, and Concord grape juice are also effective in reversing motor behavior problems in lab rats.

In addition, anthocyanins, a particular type of polyphenol antioxidant found in blueberries, have been shown to improve glucose metabolism, insulin resistance, and the functioning of a particular cell in the pancreas that's responsible for insulin production and secretion. A large study showed that a high intake of anthocyanins (particularly through the consumption of blueberries) was significantly correlated with a lower rate of type 2 diabetes.

And in several human intervention trials, blueberries and other berries significantly improved insulin sensitivity, reduced fasting blood glucose levels, and decreased postmeal spikes in blood sugar. We'll be talking a lot about controlling blood sugar throughout this book because it is probably the most important thing you can do to improve your own and your unborn child's health now and in the future.

As an ophthalmologist, I see hundreds of diabetics every year who are monitoring their eye health for diabetes-related problems. I always recommend that they have a cup of berries every day, because berries protect the blood vessels that diabetes attacks.

Animal studies are currently showing more and more ways that blueberries can affect health. In one study, hamsters whose feed was spiked with blueberry juice by-products showed a 22 to 27 percent decrease in their cholesterol levels. And studies in mice show that blueberries may play a role in reducing the formation of atherosclerotic plaques that, in humans, increase the risk for cardiovascular disease.

Particularly interesting for moms-to-be is that the health of rat mammary glands was shown to be improved in the offspring of rat mothers who had been fed 5 percent blueberry powder in their rations during pregnancy and while they were nursing. This is the first indication in animals that a mother's blueberry consumption can have an effect on the normal, healthy development of breast tissue in her offspring.

These are all exciting studies, and as they continue, I would urge everyone to consume at least a cup of berries on a daily basis. The consumption of fresh blueberries in the United States is about three times greater today than it was ten years ago.

Broccoli (and Brussels Sprouts, Red and Green Cabbage, Kale, Turnips, Cauliflower, Rutabaga, Kohlrabi, Broccoflower, Bok Choy, Collards, Mustard Greens, Turnip Greens, Swiss Chard, Arugula, Watercress, Daikon, Wasabi, and Liverwort)

Cruciferous vegetables, and broccoli in particular, are powerful anticancer foods. Broccoli contains a chemical called indole-3-carbinol that helps to reduce the effects of environmental pollutants like dioxins, which can negatively affect your hormones by preventing them from binding to the estrogen receptors in your body. Many recent reports also suggest that cruciferous vegetables are a good source of natural antioxidants because of their high levels of carotenoids, tocopherols (part of the vitamin E family), and vitamin C, all of which may help to protect the body from free radical damage.

In addition, numerous studies have shown that cruciferous vegetables contain high levels of polyphenols, which, as noted earlier, possess a myriad of health-promoting properties, especially antioxidant activity.

Broccoli contains high concentrations of quercetin, which is known to protect the body from cardiovascular disease, cancer, and cataracts. In conjunction with other nutrients, quercetin has the ability to prevent the oxidation of LDL cholesterol by neutralizing free radicals and binding with potentially toxic metals. As a result, quercetin may aid in the prevention of cancer, atherosclerosis, and chronic inflammation by retarding oxidative degradation, inducing enzymes that detoxify carcinogens, and deactivating at least thirty types of agents that may cause cancer. Kale leaves, which are also rich in quercetin and other polyphenols, have been shown to reduce the adverse effects of a number of pathogenic bacteria as well as pathogens known to cause respiratory illnesses in humans.

For cruciferous vegetables in general, the leaves (and in the case of broccoli, the florets) contain more bioactive substances than the stems do. Organic gardeners will be interested to learn that insect attacks on organically grown crucifers actually seem to *increase* the polyphenols in the crop, and the nitrogen and sulfur in organic soil are essential for a high production of polyphenols by the plant. It has also been shown that steaming is the ideal method of cooking to preserve many of the bioactive nutrients in cruciferous vegetables.

Chocolate, Dark

It may surprise you to find chocolate on anyone's list of health-promoting foods. I'm certainly not telling you to go out and consume a supersize milk chocolate bar. However, the cocoa in good-quality dark chocolate contains polyphenol antioxidants called flavonols that lower blood pressure and prevent plaque formation in the arteries. A 2008 study showed that dark chocolate (compared to white chocolate) both increased blood flow through the arteries and reduced blood pressure.

A study of hypertensive patients showed that dark chocolate not only significantly reduced blood pressure but also improved insulin sensitivity. Other researchers have found that these effects, plus a reduction in LDL cholesterol and increased HDL cholesterol, resulted from the consumption of "flavonoid-rich cocoa" rather than other forms of chocolate such as candy bars. I enjoy at least 6 grams of organic nonalkalinized cocoa five to seven days a week.

Because chocolate products are often high in sugar and fat, it is generally assumed that eating chocolate leads to weight gain. However, a study of 975 healthy men and women ages twenty to eighty-five at the University of California–San Diego School of Medicine, where I am an assistant clinical professor in the department of ophthalmology, showed that adults who consumed chocolate more frequently had lower body mass index (BMI, or weight relative to height) numbers than those who consumed it less often.

The results were not explained by calorie intake, because frequent chocolate intake was linked to more overall calories; nor were they explained by activity or any other potential factors. Although it runs counter to conventional wisdom, this finding is in accordance with a growing body of literature suggesting that the character, and not just the quantity, of calories consumed has an effect on BMI and other indicators of metabolic syndrome. Metabolic syndrome, which increases the risk of cardiovascular disease and stroke, is characterized by the International Diabetes Federation as any three of the following:

- Large waist circumference: more than thirty-five inches for women and forty inches for men, unless there is a family history of diabetes, in which case it would be thirty-one to thirty-five inches for women and thirty-seven to thirty-nine inches for men

- Triglyceride level more than 150 mg/dL
- HDL less than 40 mg/dL for men or less than 50 mg/dL for women
- Systolic blood pressure more than 130 or diastolic more than 85
- Fasting blood glucose level 100 mg/dL or higher

A recent publication reported that a particular antioxidant, cocoa-derived epicatechin, increased the growth and division of the mito-chondria (the cells' energy producers); increased capillary action, muscular performance, and lean body mass; and reduced weight without changing calories or exercise in rodents. Parallel processes in humans, if they exist, could explain the findings in the California study. The authors of that study stated the following in conclusion:

> Our findings—that more frequent chocolate intake is linked to lower BMI—are intriguing. They accord with other find-ings suggesting that diet composition, as well as calorie number, may influence BMI. They comport with reported benefits of chocolate to other elements of the MetS [meta-bolic syndrome]. Compatible experimental findings in rats given epicatechin from cocoa suggest the association could be causal. A randomized trial of chocolate for metabolic benefits in humans may be merited.

In addition, dark chocolate has been shown to protect the skin from sun damage and to increase the serotonin (a feel-good chem-ical) level in the brain—which may be why we like chocolate so much. That said, these benefits come only from good-quality dark chocolate with at least 70 percent cocoa solids.

Dried and Freeze-Dried Fruits

Because they are so concentrated, dried fruits, measured by volume, have a higher content of polyphenol antioxidants and more fiber than their fresh-fruit counterparts. You can now find almost every variety of fruit, from cherries to pears, in dried form. The most nutri-ent-dense dried fruits are apricots, figs, prunes, raisins, dates, straw-berries, blueberries, and cranberries. Just be sure the ones you buy are not sweetened with high-fructose corn syrup. And try to find organic brands, because whatever pesticides the fruit might have been sprayed with will also be concentrated when it is dried.

Extra-Virgin Olive Oil, First Cold-Pressed (and Canola Oil)

First cold-pressed extra-virgin olive oil is the highest-quality olive oil with the maximum phytonutrient content.

A study published in the journal *Nature* reported that oleocan-thal, a compound naturally occurring in extra-virgin olive oil, pre-vented the production of two proinflammatory enzymes in the same way as anti-inflammatory drugs like ibuprofen and aspirin—without the stomach problems those medications can cause. It also has the highest percentage (about 75 percent) of monounsaturated fat of any culinary oil, and studies have shown that when other dietary fats were replaced with olive oil, the participants' total cho-lesterol levels decreased, while their ratio of LDL to HDL choles-terol improved.

There is an impressive body of evidence supporting the benefits of olive oil for prevention of many chronic degenerative diseases and the aging process. It has been shown that the antioxidant poly-phenols in first cold-pressed extra-virgin olive oil not only neutral-ize free radicals but also modulate cell signaling and gene expression in various pathways. One study has shown that these polyphenols reduced the gene expression associated with atherogenic (plaque buildup) and inflammatory processes.

The authors of this study also reported a reduction in a protein whose overexpression can lead to the production of new blood ves-sels necessary for cancer growth. This is a fascinating and important example of how the foods we eat can manipulate and affect genetic expression.

Garlic

Since ancient times, garlic has been used for the treatment of disease. It has been found in Egyptian pyramids and ancient Greek temples and is one of the earlier performance-enhancing drugs, having been given to the original Olympic athletes. Garlic contains more than a hundred different nutrients and is a powerful anti-inflammatory. You can buy it in supplements, but I believe that it provides more health benefits when eaten as food.

Allicin, a sulfur compound in garlic that is responsible for its antibacterial, antiviral, and antifungal properties, is partly destroyed in cooking, but many of its other health-benefiting elements—including flavonoids, selenium, and other sulfur compounds—are not destroyed in cooking. So if you're not a lover of raw garlic, do at least use it in cooking. My favorite way to use garlic is to stir-fry it in a bit of first cold-pressed extra-virgin olive oil. For more on garlic, see chapter 3.

Honey

The flavonoids in honey help regulate blood sugar level, and the darker the honey, the more flavonoids it contains. Honey also has a high level of oligosaccharides, which promote the growth of good bacteria in the colon and thus support gastrointestinal health. Drizzle honey on yogurt and use it in salad dressings or in place of other sweeteners to gain its many health benefits.

Kiwis (as well as Strawberry Guavas, Pineapple Guavas, and Brazilian or Lemon Guavas)

Not so many years ago, kiwis were considered an exotic fruit, at least in the United States. Now they're available almost everywhere, and that's a good thing, because they're actually full of important nutrients. In fact, kiwis are an excellent source of both vitamin C and vitamin E and contain significant amounts of the carotenoid antioxidant lutein, which is good for the eyes. Kiwis have more vitamin C than an equivalent amount of oranges, and this important nutrient is the primary water-soluble antioxidant in our body, boosting our immune system and reducing the severity of problems like arthritis and asthma. Both dietary (as opposed to supplemental) vitamin C and vitamin E are good for the brain, the heart, and the eyes, having been shown to lower the rate of age-related macular degeneration and dementia. Supplement studies of these two vitamins have shown mixed results, and although I strongly support the use of supplemental vitamin C and vitamin E, I believe that it is essential also to obtain these two important nutrients from food sources.

The *British Journal of Nutrition* reported that in a study of thirty-two individuals at least sixty-five years old, the consumption of four golden kiwis per day reduced the severity and duration of head congestion and the duration of sore throat associated with upper respiratory infections. Since kiwis have the highest density of vitamin C of any fruit as well as significant amounts of vitamin E, the investigators speculated that their findings were related to increased blood levels of vitamin C and vitamin E (along with other substances).

If you rub off the brown fuzz on the surface of the kiwi, you can eat the skin, which is where many of the fruit's nutrients are stored.

Oats (and Oat Bran, Wheat Germ, Ground Flaxseed Meal, Brown Rice, Wild Rice, Barley, Wheat, Buckwheat, Rye, Millet, Bulgur Wheat, Amaranth, Quinoa, Triticale, Kamut, Yellow Corn, Spelt, and Couscous)

A 2007 review of the literature relating to the effect of whole grains on coronary heart disease in clinical intervention trials found evidence for a protective benefit limited mainly to whole-grain oats. The consumption of oatmeal or oat bran, for even short periods, has been shown in the majority of studies to reduce total and LDL cholesterol levels, which are two of the primary risk factors for coronary heart disease. In addition, oats have been shown to improve the function of the cells that line the blood vessels, when consumed with vitamin C and E, and to reduce blood pressure.

Oats contain more than twenty unique polyphenol compounds not found in other grains that have been shown in animal studies to increase the antioxidant enzyme systems in skeletal muscle, the liver, and the kidneys; to enhance the production of glutathione antioxidant enzyme systems in the skeletal muscle and the heart; and to decrease the production of free radicals during exercise.

In summary, oat consumption keeps the heart healthy by lowering total and LDL cholesterol, suppressing inflammation, relaxing arteries, and inhibiting abnormal muscle-cell growth in the vascular system. The antiproliferative effect of oats on colon cells may also reduce the risk of colon cancer. Finally, it has been known for centuries that oats have an anti-irritation effect on the skin. So if your mother told you to eat your oatmeal because it was good for you, she was right—again.

In addition to oats, all of the other whole grains are great sources of fiber, and a high-fiber diet is known to reduce inflammation, which in turn reduces the risk for many chronic diseases.

Quinoa is one of only two plant-based sources (the other is soy) of complete protein, which means that it contains all of the essential amino acids our bodies can't manufacture for themselves.

In recent years, many people have eliminated bread from their diets in order to lose weight, but not all breads are created equal, and some breads are getting a bad rap. Whole-grain bread is an important source of carbohydrates, proteins, fiber, iron, zinc, and vitamin B_1, and it contains significant quantities of potassium, magnesium, niacin, vitamin B_2, vitamin B_6, and folic acid.

A 2008 review analyzed the role of cereal grains in weight management and concluded that overall, whole-grain cereals were correlated with low BMI, low waist measurement, and a decreased rate of being overweight. The same article indicated that there is some evidence that a high intake of refined grains can cause minor increases in waist circumference in women. Epidemiological studies have clearly shown that whole-grain cereals can protect the body from obesity, cardiovascular disease, and diabetes.

The specific effects of whole grains include increased satiety, decreased glycemic response, and reduced transit time through the gastrointestinal tract. In addition, the magnesium in whole grains is essential for proper insulin action, and the wide array of anticarcinogenic, antioxidant functions of the bioactive compounds found in the germ and the bran are well recognized as protective.

In short, whole-grain bread does not appear to be correlated with weight gain, and, in fact, it may actually be beneficial to weight status in addition to its other health benefits.

Onions (and Chives, Scallions, Shallots, and Leeks)

Onions are high in flavonoid antioxidants, particularly quercetin (which was discussed under broccoli). Most of the onion's quercetin is in the outermost layer, just beneath the papery skin, so peel just enough but not too much to get the most out of your onion. Also, when you cook onions to make soup, the quercetin is not lost; it is just transferred to the liquid. Drink up!

Oranges (and Tangerines, Tangelos, Lemons, Limes, White and Pink Grapefruit, and Kumquats)

Aside from the vitamin C we all know about, oranges are rich in folate, which is particularly important for any woman who is pregnant or planning to become pregnant because of its proven ability to lower the level of homocysteine, an amino acid that, at high levels, has been correlated with numerous adverse health conditions (see chapter 5). The peel and the inner white pulp of the orange contain hesperidin, a phytonutrient that has been shown to lower blood pressure and cholesterol levels in laboratory animals. Try grating orange rind on salads or fish to get these important benefits. Or do as my mother insisted and take a bite of the skin (as long as the orange is organic and therefore hasn't been sprayed with pesticides).

Red, or blood, oranges in particular have a class of polyphenols called anthocyanins, which give the fruit its red color. One study demonstrated that drinking blood-orange juice on a daily basis rapidly improved and normalized the functioning of the cells that line the blood vessels in nondiabetic subjects with risk factors for cardiovascular disease.

Blood oranges are also high in vitamin C and carotenoids, which are also likely contributors to their favorable effect on the cells that line the blood vessels, as measured by blood flow. The same study also showed that red orange juice had a significant anti-inflammatory effect (measured by a decrease in inflammatory markers in the blood). A reduction in oxidative stress markers has also been reported for consumption of regular orange juice.

Pomegranates or Pure Pomegranate Juice (and Plums, Peaches, and Nectarines)

Pomegranates have been getting rave reviews for their many health benefits, and for good reason. They contain powerful antioxidants and anti-inflammatory chemicals, and drinking pomegranate juice has been shown to lower high blood pressure and increase blood flow throughout the body. Increased blood flow to the ears and the eyes may help to reduce hearing loss and prevent macular degeneration, both of which are relatively common diseases of aging.

The paraoxonase family of enzymes found in HDL cholesterol exert a powerful antioxidant effect on the fats contained in both HDL and LDL cholesterol and also work to keep the cells lining our blood vessels in optimum health, thereby helping both blood flow and blood pressure. It has been shown that some of the substances in pomegranates actually increase the activity of this important enzyme system.

One of the polyphenols in pomegranates has been shown to decrease our body's production of triglycerides (a fat found in the blood), and pomegranate juice also provides us with another natural way to reduce the stickiness of our platelets (the aspirin-like effect). Substances in pomegranates also help to enhance insulin sensitivity by suppressing the secretion of resistin, a compound that plays a role in obesity and type 2 diabetes.

In addition, pomegranates have shown promise in the prevention and treatment of both osteoarthritis and rheumatoid arthritis. And in laboratory models, at least, they have shown promise in the prevention and treatment of cancers of the breast, the liver, the colon, and the skin. A number of human clinical trials have also shown promising results in the prevention and treatment of prostate cancer.

Pomegranates have also shown benefits in oral health by helping to control plaque development, which leads to gum disease (gingivitis).

Even male fertility may get a boost: at least two animal studies show enhanced sperm production through the antioxidant effects of pomegranate. There are also laboratory and clinical studies suggesting that pomegranates can play a role in decreasing the incidence of trichomonas vaginalis infections, a common cause of vaginitis in women of reproductive age.

The fruit may be a bit messy to eat, but the seeds are great in salads, and the juice (pure, not blended), which you can buy, has the same benefits as the fruit itself.

Pumpkin (and Carrots; Butternut Squash; Sweet Potatoes; Orange, Red, Yellow, and Green Bell Peppers; Mangoes; and Apricots)

Mouthful for mouthful, pumpkin is the best food source of alpha- and beta-carotene (see chapter 7), and there is evidence that these particular carotenoids may play a beneficial role in reducing the risk of estrogen receptor–negative breast cancer (that is, breast cancer that does not grow in response to either the body's natural production of or orally ingested estrogen) by inhibiting the ability of free radicals to induce DNA damage, a crucial step in carcinogenesis.

These carotenoids can also be metabolized to form vitamin A, which is important for the control of cellular differentiation, cellular proliferation, and immunological functions. In one study, the women who had the highest amount of alpha-carotene had a 13 percent lower rate of estrogen receptor–negative breast cancer than those who had the least, and those who tested highest for beta-carotene had a 16 percent lower rate than those who tested lowest. In addition, according to the longevity literature, alpha- and beta-carotene are two carotenoids correlated with a biological age that is lower than actual calendar age.

The nutrients in both fresh and canned pumpkin have been shown to protect the skin from damage caused by ultraviolet light and to reduce photosensitivity. In general, the carotenoids in pumpkin are correlated with protection from cataracts and skin cancer, the promotion of lung health, and increased immune system function.

Soy (Tofu, Soy Milk, Soy Yogurt, Soy Nuts, Edamame, Tempeh, and Miso)

Like quinoa, soy is a plant-based source of complete protein, and unlike animal sources of protein, soy contains very little saturated fat.

Soy contains antioxidant polyphenols known as isoflavones, which are considered plant estrogens because of their molecular similarity to the female sex hormone estradiol, the primary estrogen manufactured by the body. Soy estrogens are highly selective; they promote the beneficial estrogen-like effects in tissues where the estrogen receptor beta predominates, but they do not provoke the harmful effects of conventional estrogen replacement therapy in tissues where the estrogen receptor alpha predominates. (The overexpression of the estrogen receptor alpha has been implicated in a number of human cancers, including endometrial, ovarian, breast, and colon.)

Soy isoflavones have been shown to play a positive, health-promoting role in reducing the rate of cardiovascular disease, preserving bone mineral density and thus helping to prevent osteoporosis, and reducing the rates of prostate, colon, breast, and recurring breast cancer. Soy also helps to prevent metabolic syndrome by reducing the risk for type 2 diabetes, lowering LDL cholesterol, improving blood sugar control, and reducing insulin resistance. The consumption of whole-food sources of soy also lowers inflammation.

Soy isoflavone molecules inhibit an enzyme involved in thyroid hormone synthesis, but this has not proved to be a problem with thyroid function in individuals who do not have a preexisting thyroid disease and who have adequate iodine intake. In 2008 the American Academy of Pediatrics stated, "There is no evidence from animal, adult human, or infant populations that dietary soy isoflavones may adversely affect human development, reproduction, or endocrine function." A couple of studies have shown that soy increased fertility problems in both male and female mice, but to date there has been no evidence that this is true in humans, and the amount of soy given to the mice in the studies would be the equivalent of pharmacological doses in humans.

For additional health benefits from soy, see chapter 3.

Spices (Cinnamon, Turmeric, Oregano, Peppercorns and many other herbs and spices)

Spice it up; variety is the spice of life! Cinnamon helps to slow gastric emptying, which means that it can reduce the effect of foods on blood sugar level. In one study, healthy individuals fed rice pudding with 6 grams of cinnamon had a significantly lower rise in their blood sugar levels (by delaying the passage of food from the stomach) after eating compared to a control group that was fed the rice pudding without cinnamon. Cinnamon has significant antioxidant properties and has been shown to reduce cholesterol levels in laboratory animals.

One of the most significant effects of dietary spices may turn out to be their ability to inhibit the oxidative degradation of fats (particularly in meats) that can occur after cooking. One study has shown that adding a rich spice mixture composed of ground cloves, cinnamon, oregano, rosemary (which is actually an herb), ginger, black pepper, paprika, and garlic powder to hamburger meat before cooking reduced the concentrations of malondialdehyde (an organic compound that results from lipid oxidation, is carcinogenic, and causes mutations) in the blood and urine after eating. In fact, spices have the highest known concentration of antioxidant and anti-inflammatory polyphenols of any commonly eaten food. These polyphenols not only inhibit the oxidation of LDL cholesterol after eating high-fat cooked foods but also stimulate the DNA repair mechanisms in the body. When possible, choose spices that say USDA organic on the label.

Spinach (and Kale, Collard Greens, Swiss Chard, Arugula, Mustard Greens, Turnip Greens, Bok Choy, Romaine Lettuce, and Seaweed)

Spinach has such a variety of health benefits that it's hard to know where to start. One cup of raw spinach contains almost 200 percent of the recommended daily value for vitamin K, which is essential for bone health. It contains beta carotene as well as lutein and zeaxanthin, both of which have been shown to reduce the risk of cataracts and macular degeneration. Spinach is also good for your brain. Animal studies have shown that it may protect the brain from oxidative stress and reduce age-related decline in brain function. And all of that is in addition to its anticancer, anti–cardiovascular disease, antiarthritis, and antidiabetes properties.

People who consume some type of leafy greens several times a week have a lower rate of diabetes, stroke, colon cancer, bone loss, maturity-related muscle loss, memory loss, cataracts, and macular degeneration than people who do not.

Tea (Green, Black, Oolong, White, and Rooibos)

Tea is an anti-inflammatory that fights the cancer-promoting effects of environmental pollutants. In addition, it has been shown to lower blood pressure, prevent cardiovascular disease, strengthen bones and gums, and boost metabolism.

The green tea polyphenols are better cancer preventive agents than the polyphenols in black tea. Studies have shown that green tea decreases the rate of hypertension, atrial fibrillation, premature death, and many cancers. Animal studies show that it prevents breast cancer in the offspring of pregnant lab animals exposed to chemicals that induce breast cancer in a fetus.

In particular, green tea provides photoprotective benefits that may be even greater when the tea is applied directly to the skin (rather than consumed as a beverage). One study has shown that green tea (either consumed or applied topically) decreases the amount of DNA damage from sun exposure. I do not recommend staying out of the sun, because some sun exposure is necessary to maintain healthy levels of vitamin D, but we need a diet full of foods like green tea (and carotenoids) that prevent sun-related immune system depression and skin cancer.

The biology of most cancers, and disease in general, begins with inflammation that subsequently develops into the disease itself, and green tea has an amazing ability to diminish both inflammation and immunosuppression. Having treated more than seven thousand skin cancers in the thirty-two years since completing my fellowship at the Massachusetts Eye and Ear Infirmary, I truly believe that the skin provides a wonderful window into overall health; in the vast majority of cases, healthy skin reflects a healthy body.

The blood level of green tea polyphenols begins to rise about twenty minutes after drinking the tea. Because dairy may decrease the absorption of green tea polyphenols, you should try to drink it between meals or with meals that do not include dairy. I also enjoy the antiwrinkle effect of green tea. My favorite green tea is Kirkland Signature Green Tea (with Matcha).

Having said all that, however, I still suggest drinking a variety of teas, because they all have unique nutrient profiles that can provide different health benefits.

Tomatoes (and Pink Grapefruit, Watermelon, Eggplant, Japanese Persimmons, Red-Fleshed Papayas, and Strawberry Guavas)

There is a tremendous and ever-expanding body of scientific literature reporting the value of consuming food sources of lycopene, especially cooked tomato products including tomato paste and tomato sauce. This is one instance in which eating a food cooked can be more beneficial than eating it raw, because lycopene only becomes highly bioavailable from tomatoes when they are cooked or processed. Cooked tomato products are the main source of lycopene in the American diet, and one of the best places to find it is tomato paste. Lycopene from fruit sources is readily bioavailable without cooking.

The Women's Health Study, with 27,261 participants, looked at four major tomato-based food products (tomatoes, tomato juice, tomato sauce, and pizza) and found that the women who consumed ten or more servings, compared to those who ate fewer than one-and-a-half servings per week, showed improvements in their total-HDL cholesterol number and in their hemoglobin A1c level (a marker for long-term blood glucose control). Another study showed an inverse relationship between the lycopene level and stiffness of the arteries—a sign of aging and vascular dysfunction—as well as between the lycopene level and C-reactive protein, a marker for inflammation.

In addition to its many antioxidant benefits, lycopene has been shown to reduce the risk of osteoporosis in postmenopausal women. Pregnant women are often encouraged to eat tomatoes to relieve the symptoms of morning sickness.

Turkey Breast, Skinless (and Skinless Chicken Breast)

There is substantial research evidence that the consumption of red meat is correlated with increased rates of cardiovascular disease (CVD), diabetes, and certain cancers. A large twenty-eight-year study followed 37,698 men from the Health Professionals Follow-Up Study and 83,644 women from the Nurses' Health Study who were free of cancer and CVD at the beginning of this study.

This research found that eating one serving per day of unprocessed red meat (beef, pork, or lamb) increased the total mortality rate during the time of the study by 13 percent, and one serving of processed red meat (such as bacon, hot dogs, sausage, salami, and bologna) increased it by 20 percent. The increase in CVD mortality was 18 percent for unprocessed red meat and 21 percent for processed meat; the increase in cancer mortality was 10 percent for unprocessed red meat and 16 percent for processed red meat.

The study concluded, "Red meat consumption is associated with an increased risk of total death, CVD and cancer mortality. Substitution of other healthy protein sources for red meat is associated with a lower mortality risk."

In addition to being one of the leanest meats on the planet, skinless turkey breast is rich in a variety of nutrients, including riboflavin, niacin, vitamins B_6 and B_{12}, iron, selenium, and zinc. Skinless chicken breast is actually higher in both saturated fat and calories than turkey breast. So if you don't want to roast a whole turkey breast, try burgers made from fresh ground white-meat turkey. Just be sure that the meat you buy is 97 percent fat-free as well as organic and from free-range turkeys, if possible.

Walnuts (and Almonds, Pistachios, Sesame Seeds, Peanuts, Pumpkin Seeds, Sunflower Seeds, Chia Seeds, Macadamia Nuts, Pecans, Hazelnuts, Pine Nuts, and Cashews)

Unless you're allergic to tree nuts, you should definitely be adding walnuts to your diet. They're great for your brain. Walnuts have the highest plant-based concentration of omega-3 essential fatty acids, which are necessary for proper brain function and to maintain the integrity of brain-cell membranes. Walnuts also have a perfect balance of omega-3 and omega-6 fats, which has been shown to decrease the incidence of cardiovascular disease.

Walnuts contain a particular form of vitamin E (gamma-tocopherol) that has been shown to protect cardiovascular health. And a recent study done at the Marshall University School of Medicine in

Huntington, West Virginia, reported in the journal *Nutrition and Cancer*, found that a modest amount of walnuts given to mice in addition to their daily diet reduced their rate of breast cancer by half.

Nuts in general have beneficial health properties. In fact, nuts, poultry, and whole grains have been shown to be three of the best foods for reducing the rates of cancer and cardiovascular disease. A six-year follow-up study of 11,895 participants found an inverse proportion of average yearly weight gain between those who did not consume nuts and those who consumed four or more servings per week. The authors of the study stated that even when the total energy (caloric) intake was slightly increased because of the addition of nuts to the diet, no significant weight gain was observed.

Several biological mechanisms may explain the lack of weight gain observed in association with nut consumption. Nuts are known to induce satiation (a feeling of fullness leading to a reduction in the total amount of food eaten in a single meal) and satiety (a feeling of fullness leading to a reduction in the frequency of meals). A 2008 study showed that 55 to 75 percent of the energy (caloric) intake from eating nuts may be compensated for by lower energy intake in future meals.

The satiation and satiety properties of nuts are attributed to the fact that they are rich in fiber and protein and also that they require significant chewing. The macronutrient content of nuts (fats, carbs, and protein) also increases the release of two gastrointestinal hormones that are associated with satiety. In addition, preliminary data suggest that the consumption of nuts might be correlated with a slight increase in the energy expended while one is at rest, or thermogenesis (the creation of heat during the burning of calories).

The incomplete mastication (too little chewing) of nuts, which is common, leads to a loss of energy-providing macronutrients—a bad idea when you're starving, but great when you're in a calorie-rich environment (as most Americans are). Finally, the monounsaturated and polyunsaturated fat in nuts is more readily utilized for energy than saturated fat or trans fatty acids, thus leading to reduced fat accumulation.

A number of studies have reported that frequent nut consumption is inversely correlated with fatal and nonfatal coronary heart disease, has a consistent cholesterol-lowering effect, and protects men from hypertension. Peanut butter has also been shown to protect women from diabetes. Pecans, walnuts, and pistachios have a high concentration of gamma-tocopherol, a form of vitamin E that is known to reduce inflammation. They have the highest concentration of total polyphenols and antioxidants, and the primary form of fat they contain is monounsaturated. All nuts are a good source of plant protein.

Pistachios are the only carotenoid-containing nuts and one of the few non–leafy green sources of lutein, which is extremely important for eye health. Pistachios have more potassium and more phytosterols (which play a role in reducing cholesterol) than any other nut and have been shown to promote heart-healthy blood lipid profiles. Studies have shown that pistachios reduce postmeal spikes in blood sugar and contribute to optimum functioning of the cells lining the blood vessels.

Almonds have shown a consistent ability to lower both LDL and total cholesterol and are rich in polyphenols (particularly in the skin), alpha-tocopherol (a type of vitamin E), the amino acid arginine, and the minerals magnesium, calcium, copper, manganese, and potassium.

Cashews have more magnesium than any other type of nut, and increasing magnesium intake by 100 milligrams per day has been shown to reduce the rate of diabetes by 14 percent. They are also the least calorie-dense of any tree nut.

Ideally, nuts and seeds should be used to replace other foods with high-energy density or unhealthy snacks. One of my favorite brown-bag lunches is a mixture of dry-roasted soy nuts (lightly salted), dry-roasted sunflower seeds, raw pumpkin seeds, dry-roasted peanuts, dates, and prunes along with a five-ounce can of Welch's 100% grape juice. It's delicious, filling, and gives me lots of energy for an afternoon of hard work.

Wild Salmon (and Alaskan or Northern Halibut, Canned Chunk Light or Albacore Tuna, Mackerel, Sardines, Herring, Trout—Wild or Farmed—Oysters and Clams—Wild or Farmed—Crab, Mussels, and Lobster)

You're going to be reading a lot about wild Alaskan salmon and other fish in this book, because I believe that fish is one of the healthiest and most beneficial protein sources you can find. Along with fruit, vegetables, nonfat organic dairy, legumes, lean poultry, and nuts and seeds, fish has been correlated with a decreased rate of cardiovascular disease.

The Amsterdam Growth and Health Longitudinal Study found that fish consumption—specifically the consumption of the omega-3 fats EPA and DHA, found abundantly in cold-water fish—was correlated with a 40 percent decrease in low-grade inflammation, independent of lifestyle risk factors and other food consumption.

EPA and DHA promote cell membrane stability, increase the production of enzymes that lead to blood vessel dilation, lower blood pressure and heart rate, and decrease the production of pro-inflammatory chemicals in the body.

Most amazing is that two servings of salmon per week, given to pregnant women starting at week twenty, have been shown to decrease blood vessel inflammation in their fetuses. This indicates that cardiovascular benefits to a baby may begin even before birth. The designers of the study stated that exposure to omega-3 in utero could possibly modulate gene expression through epigenetic changes and lead to a decreased susceptibility to atherosclerosis (and thus the development of cardiovascular disease) later in life.

Yogurt, Nonfat Organic (and Kefir, Greek Yogurt, Soy Yogurt, DanActive Immunity, and Nonfat Organic Milk)

One of the most important benefits of including yogurt in your diet is that it is a great source of probiotics, the health-promoting bacteria that keep our gastrointestinal system at peak performance in efficiently processing calories and nutrients. Nonfat organic yogurt plays a role in controlling weight and blood pressure as well as in preventing osteoporosis.

Much has been written lately about the possible relationship between the consumption of dairy products and an increased risk for various cancers, but that may be related to the hormones administered to cows to increase milk production. So look for organic dairy or at least rBGH-free dairy products.

Dairy products are the best source of calcium and a good source of protein, magnesium, the B vitamins, and vitamins A and D. In fact, studies have shown that dairy products may well protect the body from some types of cancer. Two Norwegian studies indicated that premenopausal women who had a high consumption of milk had a lower rate of breast cancer than women who had low or no milk consumption. Low-fat or nonfat dairy seems to have a better anti–breast cancer effect, and the fat from milk and butter does seem to be positively correlated with breast cancer.

The incidence of colon cancer is also reduced in subjects with high and regular consumption of dairy products, and fermented milk or yogurt seems to provide a protective effect. In a study evaluating the links between dairy product consumption and cancer, the authors concluded that "among all dairy products available, cultured milk, yogurt, and low-fat dairy products seem to be better choices for providing nutrients to prevent not only cancer but other chronic diseases as well."

Take a Multivitamin

It's best to get all of the nutrients you need from food sources first, because there is no supplement that can provide the synergy of the thousands of nutrients that nature provides in whole foods, and it is virtually impossible to get too much of a good thing from food. Having said that, however, I would also recommend that couples trying to become pregnant supplement their diet with a multivitamin.

The Nurses' Health Study and the Nurses' Health Study II are two of the largest investigations ever conducted of risk factors for major chronic diseases in women. One finding of the two studies is an inverse correlation between the frequency of multivitamin consumption and the condition of ovulatory infertility. The rate of this type of infertility was lower among women who consumed three or more multivitamins a week than among women who didn't take multivitamins.

One possible explanation for this is that the components of multivitamins, including antioxidants and folic acid, improve fertility through the reduction of oxidative stress. So even if you're following a SuperFoods diet, it can't hurt to also take a multivitamin, which could just turn out to be the icing on the cake, so to speak.

Cut Down on Caffeine and Alcohol

Most women know that alcohol and pregnancy don't mix. The reports about drinking coffee while pregnant have been conflicting. But now there are a number of studies showing that both can be detrimental to *conception*.

A 1998 study of 430 couples planning a first pregnancy showed that the women who consumed alcohol were less likely to conceive within six menstrual cycles than those who abstained. In addition, the more they drank, the longer it took for them to become pregnant. In a study of the relationship between alcohol consumption and ovulatory factor infertility, moderate drinking (fewer than seven drinks a week) seemed to create a delay in conceiving, and drinking more than seven drinks a week was correlated with a 60 percent longer time to conceive.

Although it is not entirely clear from the evidence so far exactly what level of alcohol consumption has a negative effect on fertility, it would seem to be wise to err on the side of caution: when you decide to get pregnant, stop drinking. Cutting out alcohol before you become pregnant will create a healthier environment for the fetus once you do conceive. You will, in effect, be cleaning house before the guest arrives.

In terms of caffeine, a multicenter European study of infertility and subfecundity (defined as taking nine and a half months to a year to conception) indicated that the consumption of more than 500 milligrams of caffeine (3 cups of coffee) per day correlated with a 45 percent increase in risk for subfecundity in a first pregnancy.

The current evidence doesn't seem to warrant cutting out caffeine entirely—consumption of 100 to 200 milligrams per day has not been associated with any adverse effect on fertility—but it would seem wise to keep consumption to one and one half cups (less than 200 milligrams) of coffee per day. And if you must have a soft drink, go with noncaffeinated diet drinks so that you avoid the unnecessary caffeine as well as the empty calories and the high-fructose corn syrup with which virtually all nondiet soft drinks are sweetened. (Although artificial sweeteners may pose a problem, I believe that the number of calories in a regular soda is more of a health threat than the amount of artificial sweetener in a diet soda.)

At least one study conducted in 1998 found that drinking tea (as opposed to other caffeinated beverages) *increased* the chances of conception twofold. Rooibos (red tea from South Africa) is caffeine-free and contains a variety of phytonutrients that studies have shown to be antimutagenic, anticarcinogenic, anti-inflammatory, and antiviral. It addition, it contains calcium, manganese, and fluoride, which promotes healthy teeth.

How Much Caffeine Are You Really Getting?
Energy Drinks

Jolt Endurance Shot (2 oz)	200 mg
Monster Energy Drink (16 oz)	160 mg
Redbull (8.46 oz)	80 mg
Rockstar (16 oz)	160 mg
Rockstar 2X Energy Drink (12 oz)	250 mg
Vitamin Energy (16 oz)	150 mg

Source: Environmental Nutrition 2012: 35(12); 3.

Soft Drinks (12 Ounces)

Jolt Cola	70 mg
Mountain Dew (regular or diet)	55 mg
Dr Pepper (regular or diet)	42 mg
SunKist Orange Soda	42 mg
Pepsi-Cola	38 mg
Diet Pepsi	36 mg
Coca-Cola Classic	34 mg
Barq's Root Beer	22 mg
Diet Barq's Root Beer	0 mg
Minute Maid Orange Soda	0 mg
Sprite	0 mg
7-Up	0 mg

Coffee (6-ounce cup made with Arabica beans)

Filter drip	130–189 mg (average 150)
Espresso (1.3–2 oz)	100 mg
Instant	50–130 mg
Decaffeinated (instant)	2–6 mg
Decaffeinated (prepared in coffee shops)	5–25 mg

Tea (6-ounce cup brewed for 3 minutes)

Green tea	10–15 mg
Black tea	50 mg
Rooibos (red tea)	0 mg

Bottled Iced Tea (16 Ounces)

Snapple (all varieties)	31 mg
Lipton (all varieties)	18–40 mg
Nestea (all varieties)	16–26 mg
Arizona (all varieties)	15–30 mg

Chocolate Products

Hot chocolate (mix, 6 oz)	10 mg
Chocolate milk (6 oz)	4 mg
Milk chocolate (28 g)	6 mg
Dark chocolate (28 g)	20 mg
Baking chocolate (28 g)	35 mg

Other Foods

Cocoa Puffs breakfast cereal (4 oz)	2 mg
Penguin Mints (1 mint)	7 mg
Dannon Coffee Yogurt (8 oz)	45 mg
Stonyfield Farm Cappuccino Yogurt (8 oz)	0 mg
Häagen-Dazs Coffee Ice Cream (1 cup)	58 mg
Haagen-Dazs Coffee Frozen Yogurt, fat-free (1 cup)	40 mg
Starbucks Coffee Ice Cream (1 cup)	40–60 mg
Ben & Jerry's No Fat Coffee Fudge Frozen Yogurt (1 cup)	85 mg

Source: T. Wilson and N. J. Temple, *Beverages in Nutrition and Health* (Totowa, NJ: Humana Press, 2004).

• •

Dr. Steve's Green Tea

Steep two green tea bags in four ounces of hot water for about three minutes. Squeeze the tea bags dry to extract twice the polyphenol content and add four to eight ounces of organic soy milk and a teaspoon of dark (preferably buckwheat) honey. After you've squeezed the tea bags, use the wet bags to wash your face—it's a great way to prevent wrinkles. I also like to use wet green tea bags on my skin to reduce the effects of sunburn.

• •

Green tea (caffeinated or not) is known for its antioxidant properties. Green tea is known to reduce the risk of breast cancer in women and in animal studies has been shown to protect the offspring of pregnant lab animals from breast cancer. Oolong and white tea are also excellent choices.

All tea has less than half the caffeine of coffee, so switching from coffee to tea is certainly a good idea in any case.

• •

Try Fertility Blend or FertiliTea

At least three European studies done in the 1990s showed that the herb chasteberry increased progesterone levels and improved fertility. It has also been shown to increase pregnancy rates and relieve premenstrual syndrome with no serious side effects.

In a controlled study of ninety-three women who had been unsuccessfully trying to conceive for six to thirty-six months, Fertility Blend—a nutritional supplement containing chasteberry, green tea extracts, L-arginine, vitamin E, vitamins B_6 and B_{12}, folate, iron, zinc, and selenium—was given to fifty-three women ages twenty-four to forty-two. After three months, fourteen of the fifty-three women (26 percent) were pregnant, compared to four out of forty (10 percent) in the control group. There were no significant side effects, and a number of fertility-enhancing hormonal changes were documented. Sounds like it's worth a try!

If you don't want to take a supplement, you can try FertiliTea—a natural fertility-enhancing blend of chasteberry, green tea, red raspberry, lady's mantle, nettle leaf, and peppermint leaf.

• •

Let's Talk about Weight

I know, no one wants to talk about weight. I get it. But the fact is that body composition plays an important role in fertility (for both women and men), so we need to have the subject on the table. There are small things anyone can do to lose a few pounds, get healthier, and therefore increase the chances of conceiving. For women, being underweight can also be a problem.

Being either overweight or underweight can affect hormonal patterns and menstrual cycles and thus fertility. Abdominal fat (measured by waist-to-hip ratio), in particular, appears more likely than overall BMI to decrease the likelihood of conception. (In chapter 3 I'll provide simple ways for you to determine your waist-to-hip ratio and your BMI.)

Obesity is correlated with menstrual irregularity, lack of ovulation, polycystic ovary syndrome (PCOS), and both male and female infertility. PCOS, which affects five-to-ten percent of women of childbearing age (generally ages twelve to forty-five), is a leading cause of infertility. Women with PCOS have at least some of the following symptoms/characteristics: no menstrual period, infrequent menses, and/or irregular bleeding; increased levels of male hormones; infrequent or absent ovulation; cystic ovaries; chronic pelvic pain; enlarged ovaries; obesity/weight gain; baldness or thinning hair; excess body hair; insulin resistance (overproduction of insulin/diabetes); hypertension; and acne/oily skin. A recent review of PCOS concluded that the prevention and treatment of obesity are important in the management of the disease.

Underweight women can experience hormonal imbalances that result in the cessation or the infrequent occurrence of the menstrual cycle.

In many instances, being underweight and not ovulating are related to extreme physical exercise, such as running marathons or participating in triathlons. But in most instances these women resume a normal menstrual cycle when they reduce their level of physical activity. A study of almost three thousand Norwegian women found that those who trained almost every day had an 11 percent increased rate of infertility, and among those who trained until they were completely exhausted, 24 percent reported fertility problems. However, the reported fertility problems lasted only as long as the hard training. If you are having trouble getting pregnant, cut back on the duration, intensity, and frequency of your physical activity. Of course, some level of regular exercise is healthier than none.

In chapter 3 I'll be talking much more specifically about what all women (and men) can and should do to get their weight under control before conceiving a child. No matter when you start or how much you do, every pound counts. Even walking around the block is better than not walking at all. And the really good news is that once you start eating more of the SuperFoods recommended throughout this book, you'll automatically start to lose weight almost without even thinking about it.

For Men: Improving Sperm Count

As I said earlier, there is a male factor that affects 30 to 40 percent of infertile couples. A major review study has concluded that between 1934 and 1996, there was an overall decline in sperm density of approximately 1.5 percent per year in the United States and approximately 3 percent per year in Europe and Australia.

Although the exact cause of abnormal sperm production remains unknown in approximately 50 percent of the cases, oxidative stress reportedly plays a role at least 30 percent of the time. And even though free radicals are necessary for maturation and egg fusion, excess numbers of free radicals can cause DNA damage, which is detrimental to reproductive outcomes and fertilization rates. So be sure to follow as many of my recommendations as possible in order to conceive.

One study reported the following:

Couples with relatively normal semen parameters should have sex daily for up to a week before [the] ovulation date. Especially in the context of assisted reproduction, this simple treatment may assist in improving sperm quality and ultimately achieving pregnancy. In addition, these results may mean that men play a greater role in infertility than previously suspected, and that frequent ejaculation is important for improving sperm quality, especially as men age during [their] reproductive cycles.

"Use it or lose it"thus seems to apply to reducing DNA damage to the sperm. So go to it, guys. Sounds like great therapy to me!

Eat More Antioxidant-Rich Foods

SuperFoods aren't sexist. Getting proper nutrition is as important for men as for women when trying to conceive. Oxidative stress has been identified as a factor contributing to male infertility. In a study of fertility clinic patients, a low intake of antioxidant nutrients was correlated with poor semen quality. The researchers concluded that "men who eat large amounts of meat and full-fat dairy products have a lower seminal quality than those who eat more fruit, veggies, and reduced fat dairy. . . . Among the couples with fertility problems coming into the clinic, the men with good semen quality ate more vegetables and fruits than those men with low seminal quality."

So men as well as women should increase their intake of the SuperFoods listed earlier in this chapter. Whoever's doing the cooking won't have to prepare separate meals, at least!

Glutathione, which we discussed in relation to increased fertility in women, has also been shown to increase sperm motility. It's a dark, lonely, dangerous swim those sperm have to make to connect with an egg, so it's a good idea to do what you can to make sure they're surrounded on their journey by the body's most effective missile-defense system. See the glutathione and cysteine foods lists earlier in this chapter.

Another powerful antioxidant specifically found to increase fertility in men by preventing free-radical damage to the seminal plasma is lycopene, which is easily obtained from tomatoes and tomato products, watermelon, and pink grapefruit. (See chapter 3 for a complete list of lycopene-rich foods.)

• •

Try Astaxanthin Supplements

Astaxanthin is a carotenoid nutrient with an intense red color that is produced by algae, bacteria, and fungi and is found in the flesh, skin, or outer skeletons of seafood such as crabs, crayfish, lobsters, krill, Alaskan sockeye salmon (which contains about 2.5 milligrams in just three ounces), Alaskan coho salmon (which contains about 1 milligram in three ounces), shrimp, and trout.

Astaxanthin has been shown to have a positive effect on sperm motility and fertility and prevent DNA damage. I would suggest trying to get 2 to 5 milligrams a day from food and/or a supplement, which should be from natural astaxanthin made from algae. Supplementary doses of as little as 1 milligram can significantly increase the blood level of astaxanthin when taken once a day for four weeks. Like all fat-soluble nutrients, astaxanthin supplements should be taken with a meal containing fat to ensure maximum absorption.

• •

Boost Fertility with Vitamins and Minerals

Low levels of vitamin C may lead to infertility and increased damage to the sperm's genetic material. The amount of vitamin C in seminal fluid directly reflects dietary intake, so see the list in chapter 4 of foods that will increase your intake of vitamin C. One study demonstrated significant improvements in sperm count in previously infertile but otherwise healthy men after the administration of 1,000 milligrams of vitamin C per day.

Vitamin B_{12}, which is required for cellular replication, is also important for increasing sperm count and motility. Dosages of 1,000 to 6,000 micrograms per day (the average being 1,500) have consistently shown improvements in sperm production. The recommended daily allowance for vitamin B_{12} is 2.6 micrograms per day, but no upper limit for tolerability has been set, and no toxicity has been found for this nutrient in any quantity. The food sources highest in B_{12} are fish, shellfish, and beef. If you're a vegetarian, you can get B_{12} from yogurt and eggs, but if you're a vegan, getting your B_{12} from supplements is essential.

Vitamin E is an extremely powerful fat-soluble antioxidant that prevents free radical damage when fat undergoes oxidation and may also prevent free radical damage to sperm cells. Good food sources of vitamin E are wheat germ; canola, peanut, soybean, and extra-virgin olive oils; almonds and hazelnuts; sunflower seeds; and peanut butter.

Vitamin E is actually composed of eight similar but different compounds—four tocopherols and four tocotrienols—and to receive the maximum benefit of this important nutrient, you should ideally be consuming food sources with all eight types of vitamin E on a daily basis. A daily combination of almonds, walnuts, pistachios, and wheat germ will get you close to the perfect mix.

Sources of Vitamin E

Alpha-tocopherol
- Sunflower seeds
- Safflower seed oil
- Olive oil
- Wheat germ oil
- Almonds
- Peanuts
- Wheat germ
- Avocados
- Spinach
- Broccoli
- Eggs
- Kiwis

Beta-tocopherol
- Corn oil
- Wheat germ oil
- Wheat germ

Gamma-tocopherol
- Soybean oil
- Corn oil
- Canola oil
- Peanuts
- Peanut oil
- Evening primrose oil
- Walnuts
- Pistachios
- Pecans
- Soybeans
- Corn
- Lima beans
- Chickpeas
- Northern beans
- Green peas

Delta-tocopherol
- Soybean oil
- Safflower oil
- Wheat germ oil
- Walnuts
- Pistachios
- Soybeans

Alpha-tocotrienol
- Palm oil
- Almonds
- Pistachios

- Wheat germ
- Barley
- Oats
- Brown rice

Beta-tocotrienol

- Wheat germ oil
- Wheat
- Barley

Gamma-tocotrienol

- Palm oil
- Pistachios
- Brown rice
- Corn

Delta-tocotrienol

- Palm oil

Some studies have shown that typical vitamin E supplementation is at best ineffective and at worst actually harmful to one's health, but that's because many supplements contain only one of the several types of vitamin E. If you are taking supplements, always buy those that contain a mixture of tocopherols and tocotrienols, and use natural (d-alpha-tocopherol) rather than synthetic (dl-alpha-tocopherol) vitamin E.

I also recommend that you find a supplemental source of gamma-tocopherol; you should take equal amounts of supplemental alpha- and gamma-tocopherol, because taking alpha-tocopherol in supplements without gamma-tocopherol may drive down the blood level of gamma-tocopherol, which is not a good thing.

The prostate gland and the semen contain large amounts of zinc, an essential mineral found in every cell of the body that helps with the development of sperm. Zinc deficiency is correlated with decreased testosterone level and sperm count. An adequate amount of zinc ensures sperm motility and production, and deficient levels are often found in infertile men with diminished sperm count. Several studies suggest that supplemental zinc may be helpful in treating male infertility.

It's necessary to get a steady supply of zinc through food and supplements, because the body has no specialized storage system for zinc. You can get zinc from shellfish, beef, chicken, turkey, dairy products, and sesame seeds. For a list of dietary sources of zinc, with the proper quantities, see chapter 4.

Selenium and glutathione are essential to the formation of an enzyme present in spermatids, the cells that form into sperm. Therefore, deficiencies in either substance can lead to defective sperm motility. Fish and shellfish are good sources, along with Brazil nuts, walnuts, eggs, and brown rice.

DHA, an omega-3 fatty acid found in fish oil, has been found to increase sperm tail motility—making the sperm better swimmers. For a list of dietary sources of DHA, see chapter 4. Try to consume 500 to 1,000 milligrams a day.

• •

Increase Fertility with Coenzyme Q_{10}

Coenzyme Q_{10} (CoQ_{10}) is necessary for the basic functioning of cells. CoQ_{10} levels have been reported to decrease with age and to be low in patients with some chronic diseases. Some researchers believe that CoQ_{10} supplementation can increase male fertility by decreasing free radical damage. See chapter 4 for dietary sources of CoQ_{10}.

• •

It's a long, hard passage those sperm have to make to meet up with an egg, so anything that protects them on their journey will increase a couple's chances of conception. Taurine is an amino acid–like molecule, manufactured by our bodies from cysteine or consumed from food, that functions as an antioxidant and detoxification molecule in the seminal fluid, thus making for healthier sperm.

SuperFood sources of taurine include eggs (free-range and high DHA, when possible), wild Alaskan salmon, lean beef from grass-fed cattle, and milk (preferably nonfat organic).

In at least one animal study, resveratrol (one of my favorite supernutrients) was shown to preserve optimum semen and sperm health. Although red wine is the best dietary source of resveratrol, in the context of fertility and conception I am recommending nonalcoholic sources of this important antioxidant. SuperFood sources of resveratrol include blueberries, cranberries, mulberries, peanut skins, pistachios, purple grapes, and purple grape juice.

Since there are no published safety studies on resveratrol for pregnant and breast-feeding women, I recommend supplement sources of resveratrol only for men. The maximum supplemental dose should not exceed 40 milligrams per day. See chapter 12 for information on where to get your supplements.

Weight Is Also an Issue for Guys

The global obesity rate parallels a documented decrease in male fertility. A recent analysis based on reviewing 9,779 men concluded that there is a correlation between being overweight or obese and having an abnormal sperm count. The authors of this study wrote that their findings could be the result of one or more of the following causes: (1) direct alterations of sperm production, (2) estrogen production from fat having a female-like effect in males, and (3) the accumulation of toxic compounds and fat-soluble endocrine-disruptive environmental toxins in fatty tissue.

It is therefore important for men to get their BMI to a satisfactory level in order to minimize male-factor infertility problems.

Detox Your Environment

We're going to talk a lot more about how to reduce your exposure to environmental toxins in the next chapter. For now, however, I want men to understand that air pollutants, water pollutants, and many of the products they use every day can have a negative effect on their ability to impregnate.

Several studies suggest that semen quality is declining worldwide as a result of the increased exposure in the past fifty to sixty years to endocrine disruptors, which are environmental chemicals that interfere with the synthesis, secretion, transport, binding, action, or elimination of natural hormones in the body. These disruptors may be found in water, soil, air, food, plastic containers, household products, and personal care products. Some are a result of exposure in the workplace. Among the most widely implicated offenders are organochlorines, polychlorinated biphenyls (better known as PCBs), dioxins, phthalates, pesticides, and herbicides.

Because so many of these chemicals are all around us, it's difficult to know which ones may be more dangerous than others or what the synergistic effects of multiple exposures might be. In the next chapter I'll talk about where they are most likely to be found and what all prospective parents can and should do to go as green as possible without going crazy. (My goal in this book is to help you *reduce* the stresses of conception, pregnancy, and parenting, not to increase them.)

One pollutant about which there is absolutely no controversy is exposure to both firsthand and secondhand tobacco smoke. In terms of pregnancy, we tend to focus on the effects that a woman's smoking has on her fetus. What you may not realize is that a number of studies have found that smoking also has an adverse effect on semen quality.

Another lifestyle choice you may want to consider moderating is your frequency of cell phone use. I know how dependent we've all become on our smartphones, but there have been some preliminary studies linking cell phone use to a decrease in sperm count, motility, and viability. Not all studies agree on the effects cell phones do or do not have, but I believe there's enough smoke out there to assume there might be a fire. So it's just one more thing you ought to be thinking about. At least avoid carrying your phone in your pants pocket. The farther you keep your cell phone, laptop, and iPad from your reproductive organs, the better off you will be.

Moving On

Whether or not you're worried about conceiving or are in fertility treatment, the recommendations in this chapter will benefit anyone who wants to have a child. They are intended for all prospective parents in conjunction with the other prepregnancy strategies that are laid out in the subsequent chapters. When it comes to parenthood, there is no either/or. We all need to take every step we can to ensure our own reproductive health and the health of our children throughout their lives.

2

Baby-Proof Your Environment before You Conceive

According to the Environmental Protection Agency (EPA), more than eighty-five thousand synthetic chemicals have been registered for use in the United States since World War II, with about two thousand new ones being produced every year for use in everything from personal care products to food, prescription drugs, lawn care products, and household cleaners. While many of these chemicals are safe, many others are not, and it's difficult to know just how many or how much we're being exposed to on a daily basis. Toxic levels are difficult to ascertain, and we don't know what the synergistic effect of exposure to multiple chemicals is on the body.

Back in 1962, Rachel Carson wrote in *Silent Spring*, "For the first time in the history of the world, every human being is now subjected to contact with dangerous chemicals, from the moment of conception until death. In the less than two decades of their use, the synthetic pesticides have been so thoroughly distributed through the animate and inanimate world that they occur virtually everywhere." Now, half a century later, those words are even more true than when they were written.

We all need to live in the world we've been given (or, rather, that we humans have created for ourselves), which means that it's impossible to avoid chemical exposure altogether, but there are many relatively simple things we can do to limit the number of chemicals in our homes and our daily environment and ways that we can protect ourselves from their harmful effects.

Since we know that certain chemicals have been associated with birth defects or health issues later in life in the children of women who were exposed to them during pregnancy, it simply makes sense to try to clean up your external environment before you ever become pregnant. This in turn will create a healthier internal environment for your unborn child. And, once again, the same goes for potential dads.

Get Xenophobic about Xenobiotics

A xenobiotic is any chemical compound that is foreign to a living organism (and should therefore not be found in that organism). Since we're all exposed to environmental chemicals every day, we all have some xenobiotics in our bodies. In the past, when the placenta was still considered impermeable, it was thought that the fetus would be protected from whatever chemicals were in the mother's blood. Now, of course, we know this isn't true. In fact, one study conducted by the Environmental Working Group assessed the umbilical cord blood of ten babies born in the United States. Of the 413 toxic compounds tested for, 287 were found to be present.

In another study, many more chemicals—including pharmaceuticals, pesticides, and heavy metals—were also found in infants' first stool.

Compound	Number of Compounds Tested	Number of Compounds Found	How Used, Where Found
Heavy metal mercury	1	1	Dental amalgams; present in seafood
Polycyclic aromatic hydro-carbons (PAH)	18	9	Combustion by-product from tailpipes and cigarettes
Polybrominated dioxins and furans (PBDD-F)	12	7	Contaminates of brominated fire retardants
Polychlorinated dioxins and furans (PCDD-F)	17	11	By-products of plastic production (PVC), industrial bleaching, and incineration
Perfluorinated chemicals (PFCs)	12	9	Teflon, Scotch Guard, fabric and carpet protec-tors, food wrap coatings
Chlorinated pesticides	28	21	Farmed salmon and other fat-containing foods; most now banned for use
Polybrominated diphenyl ethers (PBDEs)	46	32	Flame retardants, high in farmed salmon
Polychlorinated naphthalenes	70	50	Wood preservatives, varnishes
Polychlorinated biphenyls (PCBs)	209	147	Lubricants and insulation, high in farmed salmon; now banned worldwide

Source: Crinnion WJ. Maternal levels of xenobiotics that affect fetal development and childhood health. *Altern Med Rev* 2009; 14(3):212–222.

Some of these have been linked to health problems, including childhood and adult cancers, immune disorders, developmental delays, and alterations in reproductive tract function. And it is difficult to know how their effects may be multiplied or moderated when they are present in combination.

We'll discuss many of these chemicals and their potential effects individually, but whatever a mother-to-be is exposed to affects her unborn child, and the fewer chemicals there are in a woman's body at the time of conception, the healthier her internal environment will be when the baby takes up residence in her womb.

Beware of Bisphenol

Bisphenol, or BPA, is used to make everything from plastic water bottles and food packaging to sunglasses and CDs. It is an environmental estrogen known to be an endocrine disruptor and has been linked to reproductive disorders, obesity, abnormal brain development, and breast and prostate cancers. In January 2010 the Food and Drug Administration (FDA) announced that it was concerned about "the potential effects of BPA on the brain, behavior, and prostate gland of fetuses, infants, and young children."

Environmental estrogens are natural or artificial chemicals existing outside the body that, when consumed, act like the estrogen naturally found in the body and activate its biochemical signaling networks in ways that can be dangerous. In one study, researchers gave BPA in drinking water to a group of mice starting a week before pregnancy at levels calculated to produce concentrations that were the same as what a human mother would consume. When the mice gave birth, their offspring had four measurable blood markers indicating a substantial risk for the development of asthma. The researchers concluded that "we have to consider the possible impact of environmental estrogens on normal immune development and on the development and morbidity of immunologic diseases such as asthma."

Every year, more than six billion pounds of BPA are used in the manufacturing of epoxy resins and polycarbonate plastics, which are then used in a variety of domestic products, including the linings of food and beverage cans, water bottles, other food containers, and even baby bottles. Numerous studies have found detectable levels in a wide range of packaged foods, which means that the chemical leaches from the container into the food itself.

BPA has been correlated with intrauterine growth restriction (leading to low birth weight), and some recent studies have found that fetal and neonatal exposure may affect the child's future fertility, influence reproductive senescence (the age at which one is no longer fertile), and create male reproductive anomalies. Human studies have shown that BPA is elevated in women who have ovarian cysts or excessive growth of the uterine lining, and rat studies have shown it to be correlated with insulin resistance, a primary biochemical condition in women with polycystic ovary syndrome).

Although the "lowest observable adverse effect level" for BPA was determined in the 1980s by the National Toxicology Program of the National Institutes of Health, animal studies conducted since then have revealed significant effects from dosages below that level, particularly when fetuses and newborns are exposed.

Recently, some states have banned the use of BPA in products used by infants and small children (such as baby bottles and sippy cups); some retailers, including Walmart and Toys"R"Us, have taken baby bottles containing BPA off their shelves; and some manufacturers of baby products have voluntarily stopped using the chemical. That's all great, but it doesn't address the issue of prenatal exposure, so women who are planning to become pregnant need to take matters into their own hands.

BPA is so ubiquitous that it would be impossible to avoid it entirely, but we can at least try to limit the amount that gets into our food and drink. That means using glass or metal bottles and food storage containers instead of plastic and either limiting the use of canned foods or looking for canned goods that do not use BPA.

....

CONSUMER ALERT

According to the website Inspiration Green (http:// inspirationgreen.com/bpa-lined-cans.html), the following foods are available in cans made without BPA:

Ecofish (Henry & Lisa's): canned tuna

Eden Foods: all thirty-three of its organic beans, chili, rice and beans, refried and flavored

Hunt's: only the plain tomatoes—but a great first step!

Muir Glen: just starting to change to BPA-free cans for its tomato products

Native Factor: coconut water

Native Forest: organic coconut milk, asparagus, mushrooms, hearts of palm, and all its canned fruits

Nature's One: organic powdered baby milk

Oregon's Choice: canned tuna

Tetra-pak (aseptic containers): lined with polyethylene, not BPA. Pomi brand chopped tomatoes in tetra-paks are becoming more widely available.

Trader Joe's: its own brand of canned corn, tomatoes, beans (except baked beans), tuna fish, anchovies, poultry, beef, coconut milk, fruit (except mandarins), and vegetables (except artichokes)

Vital Choice: canned salmon, albacore tuna, sardines, and mackerel

Wild Planet: canned tuna

Whole Foods: 27 percent of its own brand of canned goods; no specifics given

PCBs May Be Banned, but They're Still with Us

Polychlorinated biphenyls (PCBs), another endocrine disruptor, were banned in the United States in 1979 because of their long-term persistence in the environment. They had been used for decades in capacitor and transformer oils, hydraulic fluids, lubricating oils, and plasticizers, and because of inadvertent spills, careless disposal, their chemical stability, and their resistance to biodegradation—in other words, their persistence—they are still with us today. Most PCBs do not mix with water, so they settle into river-beds, lake bottoms, and coastal sediments, where they bioaccumulate and enter the food chain, primarily through fish and shellfish from freshwater and coastal areas.

Studies have consistently shown that prenatal exposure to PCBs is correlated with specific cognitive impairments, including executive brain function, processing speed, verbal abilities, and visual memory.

....

CONSUMER ALERT

To reduce the risk of eating seafood contaminated with PCBs, the Environmental Defense Fund recommends the following:

- Before cooking, remove the skin, the fat (found along the back, sides, and belly), the internal organs, the tomalley (liver) of lobster, and the mustard (nonmeat portion) of crabs, where toxins are likely to accumulate.
- When cooking, be sure to let the fat drain away, and avoid or reduce the consumption of fish drippings.
- Serve less fried fish; frying seals in chemical pollutants that might be in the fish's fat, whereas grilling, sautéing, or broiling allows the fat to drain away.
- For smoked fish, it is best to fillet the fish and remove the skin *before* the fish is smoked.

  Aside from following the above tips for seafood, you should reduce your consumption of saturated animal fats in general. Choose the following instead:
- Butter substitutes (such as Smart Balance Organic Whipped Buttery Spread). If you must have butter, I recommend getting organic and unsalted. You can find organic butter at http://www.Horizonorganics.com and http://www.edenfoods.com. Many market chains, such as Von's O Organics, carry their own lines of organic dairy products.
- Wild Alaskan salmon
- Sardines

- Skinless turkey breast
- Buffalo meat (available from http://www.jhbuffalomeat .com and http://www.buffalogal.com)
- Lean meat from free-range, grass-fed animals; available from stores like Whole Foods and Trader Joe's. My favorite is Niman Ranch (http://www.nimanranch.com).

Trim all excess fat from meat and choose the leanest cuts, such as top round, eye of round, or sirloin, and stick to portions of no more than three to four ounces each. Avoid the highest saturated-fat foods, which have the highest concentration of toxins, such as high-fat cuts of beef, bacon, frankfurters, whole-milk cheeses, butter, and fatty fish (such as farm-raised salmon).

Pesticides Are Poison

The purpose of pesticide is to kill things. There are many different kinds of pesticides (and herbicides), all of which are used to kill insects, weeds, fungi, rodents, and other pests. They bring the substantial public health benefit of increasing productivity in the food industry and decreasing the incidence of disease. But they can also have serious detrimental effects on all humans (and household pets), but especially on the developing fetus. In terms of their potential effects on prenatal health, all pesticides are neurotoxins; this means that they work by attacking the brain, which controls the nervous system. In the fetal neurological system, the blood-brain barrier is still being developed, making the fetus that much more susceptible to such neurotoxins.

More than one billion pounds of pesticides are used in the Unites States every year. Of those, 71 percent are used in commercial agriculture, and 15 percent are used in homes and gardens. It is estimated that the average home contains three to ten gallons of hazardous materials. So the least we can do is try to keep these toxins out of our personal environment.

One study has shown a strong correlation between birth defects and the pesticides found in surface water (that is, streams, rivers, lakes, and oceans). The researchers studied all the births occurring in the United States between 1996 and 2002 and found an increased number of birth defects—including spina bifida (in which the bones of the spine do not form properly around the spinal cord), cleft lip, clubfoot, and Down syndrome—in babies born to women whose last menstrual period occurred in April, May, June, or July, the time of year that concentrations of pesticides in surface water are at their peak. The researchers concluded, "While our study did not prove a cause-and-effect link, the fact that birth defects and pesticides in surface water peak during the same 4 months makes us suspect that the two are related."

The three most commonly used forms of nonpersistent pesticides are organophosphates, carbamates, and pyrethroids. Organophosphates are used to control fungi, weeds, insects, and other so-called pests. They work primarily as neurotoxins, killing insects by disrupting their brains and nervous systems, and have been found to do the same thing in humans by inhibiting acetylcholinesterase, a chemical that is necessary for the proper functioning of the nervous system.

They are known to cross the placenta, and chronic exposure to organophosphates has been correlated with infertility linked to testicular cancer, poor semen quality, endometriosis, birth defects like spina bifida, hydrocephaly (excess cranial fluid resulting in an enlarged skull), shortened limbs, attention deficit/hyperactivity disorder (ADHD), and lower cognitive (IQ) scores at age seven in children exposed as fetuses.

Other findings linked to organophosphate exposure include decreased reflexes at birth, problems with short-term memory, and impaired mental development. Organophosphates have also been shown to affect the neurotransmitter serotonin and cause long-lasting changes in the brain's drug-addiction systems.

In the study mentioned earlier in this chapter that tested chemicals in infants' first stool, organophosphate metabolites were among those that were found. In addition, more than 93 percent of the children tested by the Centers for Disease Control (CDC) for its July 2005 *National Report on Human Exposure to Environmental Chemicals* had at least one detectable measure of the six organo-phosphates for which the children were tested.

Interesting to note is that the data reported thirty to forty years ago on the link between lead exposure and decreased IQ were very similar to the data linking organophosphates to ADHD. Even minor exposures can be harmful. And because there does not seem to be an effective treatment for children with elevated blood concentrations of lead, "getting the lead out" prior to conception is the ideal way to deal with this environmental contaminant. One way to do that is to eat foods that are rich in iron (see list in chapter 7) along with those that are high in vitamin C (see chapter 4). Iron is better absorbed and more bioavailable when you also have vitamin C in your meal, and when you consume more iron, you absorb less lead.

* *

Avoid the "Dirty Dozen"

Organophosphate pesticides are easily avoided simply by staying away from commercial varieties of the twelve fruits and vegetables found to have the highest degree of pesticide contamination. Buy them organic whenever possible. One study has shown that organic diets significantly reduce children's dietary exposure to organophosphates—so assumedly the same strategy will work for mothers-to-be.

Following is a list of the "dirty dozen," starting with the worst, provided by the Environmental Working Group (http://www.ewg.org):

1. Apples
2. Celery
3. Strawberries
4. Peaches

5. Spinach
6. Nectarines (imported)
7. Grapes (imported)
8. Sweet bell peppers
9. Potatoes
10. Blueberries (domestic)
11. Lettuce
12. Kale and collard greens

And here is a list of the "clean fifteen," starting with the best, that you probably don't need to buy organic:

1. Onions
2. Sweet corn
3. Pineapples
4. Avocado
5. Asparagus
6. Sweet peas
7. Mangoes
8. Eggplant
9. Cantaloupe (domestic)
10. Kiwi
11. Cabbage
12. Watermelon
13. Sweet potatoes
14. Grapefruit
15. Mushrooms

• •

Another way to evaluate pesticide risk is to use Dr. Charles Benbrook's Dietary Risk Index (DRI), which compares the average pesticide levels found on a food to the maximum levels that the U.S.

Environmental Protection Agency regards as safe. Using this methodology, the fruits highest on the DRI are peaches and nectarines from Chile, and the vegetables highest on the DRI are sweet bell peppers from Mexico, cucumbers from Honduras, green beans grown in the United States, and asparagus from Peru. This information can be found at http://www.organicconsumers.org/organics bytes.cfm or http://www.organic-center.org.

Pyrethroids are man-made pesticides similar to the natural pesticide pyrethrum, which is produced by chrysanthemums. Pyrethroids are used as household insecticides, as pet sprays and shampoos, as mosquito repellents, and to treat lice. They have also been an important tool for stopping the spread of West Nile virus.

Pyrethroids work by altering nerve function, which causes paralysis in target insect pests, eventually resulting in death.

Although pyrethroids are considered less toxic to humans than organophosphates, one study has shown that when female rats were fed very high doses of pyrethrins for three weeks prior to mating, their offspring had low body weight. In addition, the chlorinated pesticide metabolite DDE has been positively and significantly correlated with low birth weight, short length, and small head circumference. Although chlorinated pesticides have been largely banned in the United States, they continue to persist in the environment and cause an ongoing threat to health.

• •

Ten Ways to Get Rid of Pests Organically

There are several nontoxic products that can be used to get rid of a variety of household pests such as cockroaches, termites, fire ants, fleas, silverfish, and many more.

1. Try boric acid. It's an inexpensive, safe, and effective way to prevent mildew and stop the growth of mold. It has antibacterial/antifungal properties and kills cockroaches, fleas, ants, and silverfish.

2. Catnip repels (but does not kill) cockroaches, ants, aphids, and rabbits, according to the American Chemical Association. Leave it out in little bags or make "catnip tea" and spray it around the baseboards and behind your kitchen counters. (*Warning:* Don't try this if you have cats!)

3. Put eucalyptus leaves or oil in drawers and closets and around houseplants. This is a trick my mother taught me. Apparently insects hate the strong odor.

4. My friend Amy, who claims to be a "mosquito magnet," places cups of water mixed with distilled white vinegar around the plants in her backyard. She says it attracts the mosquitoes so that they leave humans alone.

5. Use organic pesticides such as Dr. Earth Pro-Active Fruit and Vegetable Insect Spray, Pro-Active House and Garden Plants Insect Spray (see http://www.drearth.com), or Concern Garden Defense Multi-Purpose Spray (http://www.arbico-organics.com).

6. Try organic fertilizers such as those made by Dr. Earth (http://www.drearth.com), E. B. Stone (http://www.ebstone.com), or BioFlora (http://www.bioflora.com).

7. Peppermint oil (the kind for external use, not the food flavoring) keeps mice away.

8. Stuff dog hair down gopher holes and spread it around tree trunks. Attach bags of dog hair to tree branches to repel gophers and ground squirrels.

9. Spray a mixture of vegetable oil and cayenne pepper onto plant/tree foliage also to repel ground squirrels.

10. "Used" cat litter, coffee grounds, and dryer sheets can also be put into gopher runs to encourage them to "go elsewhere."

Stop Smoking!

Of course you know that you should have stopped smoking a long time ago. But if you haven't, now's the time to do it. And I don't mean just prospective moms; the dads need to stop, too. In terms of your own health, smoking is the number one preventable cause of age-related macular degeneration and is estimated to be a significant factor in at least 20 percent of cataracts. In addition, it decreases the blood levels of lycopene, vitamin E, beta-carotene, lutein, zeaxanthin, beta-cryptoxanthin (one of the six carotenoids eaten by humans, and that our body can convert to vitamin A), vitamin C, and vitamin A.

Secondhand smoke has been linked to increased rates of asthma, chronic lung disease, lung cancer, and cardiovascular disease. We know how harmful secondhand smoke is for children, but babies can also be exposed before birth. And studies show that even if the mother doesn't smoke herself but is exposed to secondhand smoke, that too can affect her unborn child.

Fetal development during the last half of pregnancy depends partly on maternal metabolic adjustments detected by the placental hormones and the subsequent oxygen and nutrient supply, and researchers believe that exposure to tobacco and tobacco smoke may affect the amount of oxygen that reaches the unborn child (because the mother's hemoglobin is poorly oxygenated). Nicotine can also cause narrowing of the blood vessels (vasoconstriction) and reduce the oxygen supply through that mechanism as well. Therefore, the researchers speculate that even apparently healthy newborns of passive smokers (nonsmokers who are exposed to secondhand smoke) may suffer subtle effects from reduced oxygen levels during the pregnancy.

People who smoke build up antioxidant defense mechanisms against the free radicals created by their smoking, but those who don't smoke do not have the same protection. Those exposed to secondhand smoke may therefore be even more at risk from the smoke than the person who is doing the smoking!

Increased rates of sudden infant death syndrome (SIDS) have been correlated not only with the mother smoking during pregnancy but also with her being exposed to secondhand smoke during pregnancy.

In another study, self-reported environmental tobacco smoke was associated with decreased head circumference. There was a significant interaction between the tobacco itself and the chemicals found in cigarette smoke, so that combined exposure had a significant multiplicative effect on birth weight and head circumference.

In addition—and in case you think it's okay to smoke pot—it has been shown that prenatal and/or perinatal THC (the principal psychoactive component of cannabis)/marijuana exposure modifies brain development and function and has a significant negative effect on school-age intellectual development.

• •

Get Some Houseplants

Humans are genetically programmed to love nature, so an easy, natural, and attractive way to detoxify your home is to buy a few houseplants, many of which absorb airborne chemicals that are harmful to humans. According to *Organic Gardening*, these are the most effective air-cleaning plants:

Areca palm

Australian sword fern

Boston fern

Bromeliads

Dracaena

Dwarf date palm

English ivy

Peace lily

Pothos

Reed palm

Rubber plant

Weeping fig

Ideally, you should have two or three plants per hundred square feet of space. In particular, keep them close to where you sit, work, and sleep.

Before you bring a plant home, ask the people at the nursery whether it has been sprayed with pesticides. They might not know, but it can't hurt to ask.

• •

Go Green without Going Crazy

There are many environmental toxins we can't avoid, such as the air pollution created by burning fuel. In fact, according to the American Lung Association, metropolitan areas in my home state of California have some of the worst ozone pollution in the country. I can't make myself crazy about that, but I can try to avoid the environmental toxins that really are avoidable. It's a lifestyle choice I've made for myself, and one that you should make, too—for your own health, for the health of your present and future children, and for the human race in general.

Two recent articles point out some of the very real problems with air pollution and our health. There seems to be a correlation between long-term exposure to air pollution and cognitive decline in older women as well as an increased rate of stroke in both men and women within hours of exposure to levels of air pollution generally considered "safe" by the EPA. We should all do whatever we can to reduce air pollution, since it seems likely that this every-day exposure is having at least as much of an effect on our children (though possibly different, cumulative, and not yet well documented).

In the next chapter we'll talk about how you can make dietary changes that will eliminate toxins from your system and protect you from the effects of those you can't avoid. Making simple changes in your diet and exercise routine will ensure that your body will provide as healthy an environment as possible for your baby when you do become pregnant.

• •

An Air Pollution Paradox

It may seem counterintuitive if your area has a significant level of air pollution, but I suggest that you sleep with a window open in seasonable weather, and whenever you get in your car, roll down the window for a few minutes. However bad the outside air may be, it's better than whatever toxins have accumulated inside the closed space. "Fresh air" is indeed still (relatively) fresh.

• •

3

Prepare Your Body
for Baby

According to the 2001–2004 National Health and Nutrition Examination Survey (NHANES) of 16,338 people in the United States, more than 90 percent of women ages nineteen to thirty had usual intakes below the government's recommended levels for fruits, several vegetable subgroups, whole grains, and milk. Of the thirteen food groups tested, dark leafy greens, orange vegetables, legumes, and whole grains had the worst showing, with almost everyone failing to meet the recommendations.

If you've been following the advice in the previous two chapters, you've already begun to ensure that you don't fall into that category. Go back to chapter 1 and recheck the list of SuperFoods to be sure you are on your way to creating a healthy internal environment that will help your baby to thrive. Keep it up! And read on to learn how to be sure that you will be as healthy as possible when conception occurs.

Take a Few Simple Tests

Each of us has specific health issues to address with a health-care professional, but there are also a few medical assessments that I would suggest *all* men and women make when they decide to start a family.

Vitamin D Level

Your doctor can order a 25-hydroxy vitamin D test. The ideal level is between 50 and 80 ng/mL.

Recent studies have shown a high level of vitamin D deficiency across all age groups and all populations throughout the world. Vitamin D deficiency in pregnant women residing in northern latitudes has been reported to range between 21 and 50 percent, and an even larger number of women have a vitamin D insufficiency (which is not as serious as a deficiency). One reason for this may be that we are becoming more careful about exposing our skin to sunlight. As a result, while we are certainly protecting ourselves from premature skin aging, wrinkles, and skin cancer, we are no longer getting the benefits sunshine can bring, because sunscreen prevents the production of vitamin D.

Being significantly overweight also prevents vitamin D from being available for use by your body. Normally, fat-soluble vitamins are stored in fat tissue and released as we need them, but when there is too much fat, we're unable to get them out of storage.

Yet even as we are getting less vitamin D, we are also finding out more about how its deficiency affects our health. Vitamin D deficiency has been correlated with an increased rate of various types of cancer, rheumatoid arthritis, type 1 and type 2 diabetes, osteoporosis, multiple sclerosis, Parkinson's disease, fibromyalgia, hypertension, age-related macular degeneration, and heart disease, among others.

Vitamin D boosts the immune system, lowers blood sugar, and maintains a healthy blood pressure, all of which are extremely important during pregnancy. It also decreases inflammation, improves muscle strength, enhances calcium intake, and plays a major role in fetal development.

Both vitamin D and calcium are needed to fully mineralize the developing skeleton, and insufficiencies of these important nutrients may limit fetal bone growth and mineralization. Low maternal vitamin D status during pregnancy has been linked to decreased infant birth weight and adverse neonatal bone conditions, including impaired fetal femoral (thigh) bone development, reduced bone mineral content, and reduced bone density.

In addition, alterations in utero may affect subsequent pediatric bone mineralization, because children whose mothers had low-serum vitamin D status during pregnancy were found to have low bone mineral content at nine years of age. Maternal calcium intake also affects fetal skeletal development. In studies of pregnant adolescents, maternal dairy product intake was positively correlated with increased fetal thigh bone length, and milk intake was correlated with an infant's total body calcium. For good sources of calcium, see chapter 7.

In studies of adults, the mother's milk and vitamin D intake were significantly associated with infant birth weight, and the mother's milk intake during pregnancy has also been linked to the subsequent spinal bone-mineral density of her child at sixteen years of age. In food-based calcium supplementation studies, it has been difficult to distinguish whether it is the calcium, the vitamin D, or other components of dairy products that are affecting neonatal bone conditions. So both calcium intake and vitamin D status should be considered important in maximizing fetal bone growth.

Finally, there is growing evidence linking a pregnant woman's vitamin D level to her child's risk of developing multiple sclerosis later in life. So getting enough vitamin D may protect your child's health years down the road.

If you live north of an imaginary line drawn from Los Angeles to Philadelphia, your skin cannot manufacture any vitamin D from sunlight during a substantial portion of the year, from sometime in November until late March or early April. In the summer months, people with pale white skin can manufacture about 20,000 international units (IU) of vitamin D from exposing their arms and legs to full sunlight for approximately twenty minutes, but dark-skinned people can make only about 5,000 IU from the same amount of exposure; this is one reason that dark-skinned people are more likely to be deficient in this important nutrient. In my practice, I have found that it is rare for my dark-skinned patients to have an adequate level of vitamin D.

Therefore, in addition to people getting some sun exposure, I recommend taking a daily vitamin D_3 supplement and eating foods that contain vitamin D. Vitamin D_2 is a synthetic vitamin, often added to foods labeled "fortified," and is only half as bioavailable as vitamin D_3.

Once you've obtained the results of your vitamin D test, ask your health-care professional to recommend how much supplemental vitamin D_3 you should be taking on a daily basis. Then recheck your level in three months.

To boost your level of this important vitamin, get out in the sunshine during the summer for at least ten minutes—ideally before 10 a.m. or after 3 p.m. when the UVB radiation is not so intense—at least three to four times a week, if not daily. Wear sunscreen on your face and ears, but let the sun shine unblocked on as much of the rest of your body as possible to get the benefits. Eat the foods listed in chapter 4 that are rich in vitamin D.

Fasting Blood Sugar Level

The fasting blood sugar level test measures your blood sugar level after you have not eaten for ten to twelve hours.

The ideal number is between 70 and 100 mg/dL. A level of 100 to 125 mg/dL indicates prediabetes, and a level of 125 or higher may indicate full-blown diabetes.

Because diabetes has long been known as a risk factor for birth defects and adverse pregnancy events, it's important for women who want to become pregnant to know in advance whether they have diabetes or prediabetes so that they can get their blood sugar under control before conception and therefore decrease that risk.

In some instances, the link between obesity and birth defects could be related to undiagnosed diabetes, because obesity and diabetes often go hand in hand.

Hemoglobin A1c

A1c is a form of hemoglobin (the oxygen-carrying pigment in red blood cells) that is measured to obtain the average plasma glucose concentration for a period of a few months.

The hemoglobin A1c test serves as a marker of your average blood glucose level for the two months before testing. A normal level of glucose produces a normal amount of what is called glycosylated hemoglobin. The percentage of glycosylated hemoglobin rises as the blood glucose level rises. Therefore, the more A1c you have, the less efficiently you are processing sugar and the more likely you are to be either prediabetic or to actually have diabetes. People who are not diabetic should aim for a level between 4 and 6 percent. Since red blood cells survive in the blood for about four months, the test is a good indicator of your average blood sugar level for the past several months.

Done in conjunction with the fasting blood sugar level test, the A1c will give you a very clear picture of whether you are prediabetic or have diabetes. Studies show that being diabetic is linked to numerous complications for both mother and fetus, which means that it is extremely important to get your blood sugar under control before conception.

A study done in Germany showed that babies who were breast-fed by diabetic mothers during their first weeks of life had a greater risk of being overweight at two years of age than babies who received donor human milk from nondiabetic women. A study published in the journal *Pediatrics* in 2012 indicated a link in children between experiencing developmental delays or being diagnosed on the autism spectrum and being born to diabetic mothers.

Although the causes of autism spectrum disorders are still unknown, it appears that maternal metabolic conditions are broadly correlated with children's neurodevelopmental problems. Furthermore, we know that diabetes is associated with obesity and that autism spectrum disorders appear to be on the rise at the same time that obesity is increasing. In the United States, almost 60 percent of women of childbearing age (defined as twenty to thirty-nine) are overweight, 33 percent of this same group are obese, and 16 percent have metabolic syndrome.

Resting Blood Pressure

About one-third of the U.S. population has hypertension (high blood pressure), and because this life-threatening condition has no symptoms, people are often unaware of its presence.

High blood pressure puts both the expectant mother and her unborn child at risk. It reduces blood flow to the placenta, thereby depriving the baby of oxygen and nutrients, which often results in low birth weight. Most seriously, the mother-to-be may develop a condition called preeclampsia, a condition characterized by high blood pressure and protein in the urine that generally occurs after the twentieth week of pregnancy. This often requires that the baby be delivered early, and it can also put the mother at increased risk for cardiovascular disease later in life.

Since there are no symptoms, getting tested is the best way to ensure that your blood pressure is under control before you get pregnant. The ideal reading is less than 120 (systolic) over 80 (diastolic); a reading between 120 over 80 and 140 over 90 is classified as prehypertension, and anything higher than 140 over 90 is hypertension.

C-Reactive Protein

C-reactive protein is a type of protein whose blood level rises in reaction to an infection or inflammation.

The ideal C-reactive protein level is less than 1 mg/dL. Anything above that indicates some degree of inflammation or infection, and when you are in a proinflammatory state, you are putting yourself and your fetus at risk. Therefore, it's wise to reduce inflammation before you become pregnant. If your C-reactive protein level is high, recheck it at least once, because it can vary.

If you have an infection, such as a cold or the flu, your C-reactive protein level will be elevated. To get an accurate assessment of inflammation, you need to have this blood test when you are healthy and not suffering any acute illness.

If you do have inflammation, there are a number of simple nutritional and lifestyle fixes to help lower it.

- Enjoy a three-and-a-half-ounce serving of fresh, frozen, or canned fish that is high in omega-3 fatty acids three to four times a week. My favorites are wild Alaskan sockeye salmon, sardines packed in extra-virgin olive oil or tomato sauce, herring, and, for men only (because of potential adverse fetal interaction), a maximum of one six-ounce can of water-packed albacore tuna per week, which counts as two servings. Also, women should have one or two 1,200 mg omega-3 fish oil capsules (1,000–1,200 mg/capsule) a day, and men should have three or four daily. For a list of foods rich in omega-3 and their portion sizes, see chapter 4.
- Two tablespoons a day of organic (if possible) ground flaxseed meal or chia seeds, both of which are rich in alpha-linolenic acid; see chapter 11 for brands.
- One cup a day of berries, all of which are extremely high in antioxidants that prevent oxidative stress and its associated inflammation; or one cup daily of cherries or purple grapes;

or four to eight ounces of pure juice from these fruits or pomegranate juice with your meals

- One to one and a half ounces of walnuts, cashews, almonds, pecans, or pistachios—raw or dry-roasted, with no added salt or oil—five times a week
- Two tablespoons a day of first cold-pressed extra-virgin olive oil in recipes, on salads, or (my favorite) on whole-wheat toast; add balsamic vinegar for flavor, as an aid to digestion, and to increase the bioavailability of other nutrients.
- No more than 100 calories of dark chocolate every day—100 percent nonalkanized chocolate is best; otherwise, be sure it is 70 percent or more cocoa solids. (Read the label!)
- More fiber: fiber is full of naturally occurring anti-inflammatory phytonutrients, and studies have shown that a diet high in fiber can reduce the C-reactive protein level. So eat lots of fruits and vegetables (which are good for many reasons), beans (which are also the best source of folate on the planet), and whole grains.
- More carotenoids! (see chapter 7)
- Spices and herbs (see chapter 1)
- Prebiotics and probiotics every day
- A 10 percent decrease in BMI if it is 25 or greater
- More foods that contain choline and betaine (see chapter 7)
- At least thirty, but preferably sixty to ninety, minutes of moderate physical activity on most days
- Seven to eight hours a night of good-quality sleep

• •

Some Facts about Fiber

Some studies have shown that too much fiber can be associated with lower hormone concentrations and a higher rate of anovulation (lack of ovulation). But in one of those studies, the authors stated that "grain and vegetable fiber were not significantly associated with anovulation." And the larger problem for most Americans is that we don't eat *enough* fiber. The current recommendations of the American Heart Association, the U.S. Department of Agriculture (USDA), and the Institute of Medicine suggest that individuals should consume 20 to 35 grams of fiber a day, depending on their caloric intake. The average fiber intake level in the United States is substantially below those levels: 13.8 grams per day for women of reproductive age.

So don't be afraid of fiber, especially if you get it from whole-food sources (rather than Metamusil or fiber supplements). Foods that are high in fiber are also generally full of other important vitamins, minerals, and antioxidant-rich phytonutrients.

• •

Complete Blood Count

The complete blood count (CBC) test will rule out anemia. Iron-deficiency anemia is the number one nutrient deficiency worldwide.

Spectracell Laboratories Nutrient Profile

Suggested nutrient profile tests are the Comprehensive Nutrient Panel, which measures thirty-three vitamins, minerals, amino acids, and antioxidants as well as carbohydrate metabolism, fatty acids, and metabolites; and the HS-Omega-3 Index, which measures the percentage of EPA and DHA in red blood cell membranes. The results of these tests should be discussed with your health-care professional. Although the tests are optional, the information will give you a clear idea of where you are, nutritionally, before conception. Many insurance companies cover part or all of the expense of these tests. (For information, call 1-800-227-5227 or e-mail Spec1@spectracell.com.)

The Body's Environmental Toxicity Load

Contact Metametrix Clinical Laboratory (http://www.metametrix .com or 800-221-4640) to inquire about being tested for porphyrins, PCBs, chlorinated pesticides, organophosphates, phthalates, parabens, BPA, volatile solvents, and heavy metals. These substances are identified by blood and urine tests. Ideally, you would like to know the results of these tests before conception so you can follow the detoxification recommendations in the next section to decrease your body's burden of these chemicals.

Three excellent websites for information on the human exposure to environmental toxins are http://www.Everydayexposures .com, http://www.ewg.org/sites/bodyburden1/es.php, and http: //www.crinnionmedical.com.

Detox through Diet

In the previous chapter we discussed a variety of environmental pollutants that can have dangerous consequences for everyone, but especially for the developing fetus. In general, the risk for an adverse effect from exposure to environmental toxins is calculated as individual susceptibility times lifetime exposure times toxic potential of the environmental exposure times synergy plus the effect of other toxins. Let your health-care professional or the counselors at a laboratory like Metametrix (http://www.metametrix.com) make these calculations for you. The fetus and the newborn are at greatest risk because their detoxification systems are not yet developed. (We are what we drink, eat, touch, and breathe but cannot eliminate.) Therefore, the best thing any woman can do to protect her own health and that of her child is to get as many toxins as possible out of her system before she conceives.

We all possess what are called phase 1 and phase 2 detoxification systems, which have to be activated simultaneously because some of the phase 1 metabolites (substances essential for metabolism) can be toxic if they are not further processed by the phase 2 system. All tissues have some ability to activate the phase 1 and phase 2 detoxification systems, but the number one detoxification organ is the liver. Relatively high detoxification capacity is also found in the gastrointestinal tract, the lungs, the kidneys, and the skin.

Although some toxins are water-soluble and require minimal processing before being eliminated in the stool, the sweat, the breath, or the urine, the majority of persistent organic pollutants (POPs) are stored in adipose tissue (fat cells). So one way to get them out of the system is to get rid of some of that fat.

If you need to lose weight, the best time is before pregnancy, because as you mobilize your fat to be burned in the weight-loss process, this also mobilizes the toxins in your fat back into circulation. Thus, when you're losing weight is also when your circulatory levels of fat-soluble toxins rise. That's why you need to have your phase 1 and 2 detoxification systems activated to rid your body of these substances.

Several studies have shown that some simple dietary changes can help to mobilize dioxins and PCBs (both of which are POPs) out of the system and prevent new ones from entering. A primary phase 1 activator is chlorophyll, which is found in abundance in green leafy vegetables such as spinach, kale, Swiss chard, mustard greens, turnip greens, and, to a lesser extent, romaine lettuce and other salad greens. One study indicated that consuming roughly 10 percent of one's diet in the form of either spinach or seaweed could increase fecal excretion of various toxins by 40 to 80 percent.

The primary phase 2 activators, in order of potency from highest to lowest, are as follows:

1. Sulforaphane, found in broccoli seeds (sprouted) and broccoli florets; the sprouted broccoli seeds may be as much as a hundred times more potent than the broccoli florets in the activation process.

2. Pinostrobin, found in buckwheat honey and, to a lesser degree, in other honey; buckwheat honey can be found in many local markets, at http://www.localharvest.org/buckwheat-honey-C5192, or at http://www.info.com/WhereToBuyBuckwheatHoney. When buying honey, look for local sources and preferably glass containers.

3. Broccoli, fresh or frozen

4. Zeaxanthin (see chapter 4)

5. Quercetin, found (in order of most to least) in red onion, yellow onion, apple skin, cranberries, blueberries, tea, broccoli, buckwheat, and cilantro

6. Curcumin, found in turmeric and cumin

7. Beta-carotene (see chapter 7)

8. Lutein (see chapter 4)

9. Lycopene (see chapter 4)

10. Chlorophyll (see above)

11. Vitamin B_{12} (see chapter 4)

12. Alpha-carotene (see chapter 7)

Other detoxification nutrients include some of the other B vitamins (B_1, B_2, and B_6), magnesium, choline, green tea (especially Matcha green tea), N-acetylcysteine, vitamin C, rice bran (7 to 10.5 grams daily), whey protein powder (partially hydrolyzed and rBGH-free), seaweed (nori, wakame), probiotics, and vitamin E.

For food sources of vitamin B_2 (riboflavin) and vitamin B_6 (pyridoxine), see chapters 7 and 4, respectively.

Vitamin B_1 (thiamine) is an important coenzyme for energy production and is concentrated in nerve and muscle cells. Thiamine deficiency (beriberi) affects the cardiovascular, nervous, and muscular systems and the gastrointestinal tract. Among the foods richest in thiamine are sunflower seeds, peas, and beans. For a complete list, with recommended quantities, see chapter 4.

Cofactors for phase 2 detoxification include the amino acids glycine and glutamine (whey protein is an excellent source), the amino acid–like nutrient taurine (see chapter 1), vitamin B_5 (pantothenic acid), magnesium (see chapter 7), and the methyl donors choline (see chapter 7), folate (see chapter 4), vitamin B_{12}, and vitamin B_6.

Glutamine is the most common amino acid in the body and is involved in more metabolic processes than any other. It serves as a source of fuel for our muscles, stimulates glutathione production, provides building blocks for the formation of genetic material (DNA and RNA), aids in the synthesis of glycogen (the form of glucose stored in our muscles), supports gastrointestinal health, and maintains the integrity and health of the cells lining our intestines. The gastrointestinal tract is one of the most important ways we eliminate toxins.

Whey protein is the best source of glutamine. Other sources are yogurt (nonfat, preferably organic), cabbage, beets, turkey and chicken breast, Alaskan sockeye salmon (and other Alaskan fish), and lean beef (preferably from grass-fed cattle). Consumption of glutamine from food sources alone is not known to cause any harmful effects.

Vitamin B_5 (pantothenic acid) is essential for a variety of chemical reactions that sustain life. It is found in foods such as corn, sweet potatoes, mushrooms, and yogurt. For a complete list, including recommended quantities, see chapter 4.

As you're detoxing your body from the POPs, you'll also want to reduce the number of new toxins you take in and protect yourself from the harmful effects of those that do slip through. Since most POPs enter the body through food, it's important to reduce your intake of the foods in which they're known to take up residence. And since they accumulate in human fat, it shouldn't be surprising that they also get stored in animal fat—specifically the white saturated fat of beef from grain-fed cattle and the skin (which contains most of the fat) of poultry. So cutting back on animal fat will also cut back your POP consumption.

The main dietary sources of dioxins (one of the most prevalent and potentially dangerous POPs) are, in descending order, beef, dairy, chicken, pork, fish, and eggs.

Seven Protective SuperFoods

Although detoxing is important, you also need to increase your consumption of the SuperFoods that protect you from the harmful effects of the toxins we can't avoid. Of the twenty-five food categories listed in chapter 1, seven are the most important for this:

1. **Soy.** Soy is a protease inhibitor, which means that it plays a role in healthy cell regulation: it inhibits chemical carcinogens (such as industrial pollutants) from being activated. Soy also contains phytoestrogens that bind to the estrogen receptors on the cells, providing your body with all the benefits of estrogen while helping to block the adverse effects of endocrine disruptors. There is no evidence that fertility is a problem in Asia, where soy consumption is high.

2. **Apples (and pears, bananas, and pineapple).** Apple consumption promotes the expression and activity of our important detoxification enzyme systems and protects our DNA from a variety of chemical exposures resulting from modern life. In addition, apples and natural, unfiltered (preferably organic) apple juice contain high levels of the antioxidant quercetin, which may protect the lungs from the harmful effects of atmospheric pollutants (including cigarette smoke) and lower one's risk of lung cancer. One study found that children who drank apple juice at least once a day were half as likely to suffer from wheezing as those who drank it less that once a month.

3. **Tea.** A 2003 Harvard study found that tea acts as a sort of natural vaccine that teaches the immune cells to recognize

invading toxins. Therefore, it can help us fight off foreign invaders in a toxic environment.

4. **Onions (and chives, scallions, shallots, and leeks).** Onions boost the phase 2 detoxification enzyme system described above.

5. **Garlic.** In animal studies, oral administrations of garlic preparations increased the activity of phase 2 biotransformation enzymes in a number of tissues. No adverse effects on pregnancy outcomes have been reported as a result of including garlic in the mother's diet. The safety of taking garlic supplements during pregnancy has not been established; therefore, I do not recommend them.

6. **Broccoli (and Brussels sprouts, red and green cabbage, kale, turnips, cauliflower, rutabaga, kohlrabi, broccoflower, bok choy, collards, mustard greens, turnip greens, Swiss chard, arugula, watercress, daikon, wasabi, and liverwort).** Like soy, broccoli helps to reduce the effects of pollutants on your hormones by blocking them from binding with estrogen receptors on the surface of your cells. In addition, broccoli is the number one food for increasing the phase 2 biotransformation enzyme system.

7. **Spices.** All spices are potent anti-inflammatories, and the most potent of all is turmeric, because it contains curcumin (which gives it its gold color), a natural detoxifier that protects the liver from the damaging effects of alcohol, toxic chemicals, and some pharmaceuticals and also helps to reduce oxidative stress. Unlike garlic supplements, curcumin supplements may be taken during pregnancy. It is known to be safe in dietary quantities up to 8 grams a day, and the average person in India consumes at least 2 grams on most days. Other SuperFood favorite spices are anise, black pepper, caraway, cayenne, cinnamon, coriander, cumin, fennel, fenugreek, ginger, licorice, marjoram, nutmeg, oregano, rosemary, saffron, sage, and thyme.

Be Sure to Get All the Vitamins and Minerals You Need

We all need a variety of vitamins and minerals to keep us healthy, but there are a few that are especially important for having a super-healthy baby.

Folate and/or Folic Acid

Folate (the form naturally found in foods) or folic acid (the man-made form found in supplements) is the B_9 vitamin, which plays a role in cell production and division, including the production of red blood cells. Folate is possibly the most important vitamin for any woman planning to become pregnant, because its lack has been strongly correlated with serious neural tube defects (NTDs), including spina bifida and anencephaly (in which parts of the brain and skull are missing), as well as premature birth, low birth weight, and miscarriage.

According to the CDC, folic acid can reduce the incidence of NTDs by as much as 70 percent. However, it is currently estimated that only between 31 and 37 percent of women of childbearing age in the United States begin folate supplementation before conception.

For SuperFood sources of folate with their quantities, see chapter 4.

Vitamin B_6

Vitamin B_6 is necessary for the synthesis of serotonin and norepinephrine (two neurotransmitters associated with stress reduction) and for the formation of myelin (an insulating layer that forms around the nerves, including those in the brain and the spinal cord). Vitamin B_6 may work with vitamin B_{12} (see below) and folate to prevent neural tube defects. Foods rich in vitamin B_6 include tuna, salmon, chickpeas, and bananas. You'll find a complete list, with the proper quantities, in chapter 4.

....

CONSUMER ALERT

Low-dose oral contraceptives can have a negative effect on the body's stores of vitamin B_6, so when women discontinue their birth control pills, they may have a B_6 deficiency to make up for. If you've been taking oral contraceptives before trying to become pregnant, it is important that you now make sure you're eating plenty of foods that are high in this important vitamin.

....

Vitamin B_{12}

Along with folate and vitamin B_6, vitamin B_{12} is necessary for the proper functioning of the nervous system and for the production of red blood cells. At least one study has shown that women with the lowest levels of vitamin B_{12} had five times the rate of giving birth to a child with an NTD than women with the highest levels. And, as with folate and other essential vitamins and minerals, if you wait until you become pregnant, when your growing baby is sharing the supplies on hand, so to speak, it will be more difficult to build to an optimal level.

Biotin

Biotin, the B_7 vitamin, is essential for at least four metabolic reactions and seems to play a role in DNA replication and transcription. Marginal biotin deficiency is relatively common during pregnancy, and a biotin deficiency has been shown to cause birth defects in several animal studies. Therefore, it would be wise to ensure that you're getting an adequate supply before you become pregnant. For a list of biotin-rich foods with the proper quantities, see chapter 4.

Iodine

Iodine is a mineral usually found in sea salt, iodized salt, and bread that contains iodized salt. Pregnant women need adequate supplies of iodine because it is essential for the baby's neurocognitive development. Approximately 38 percent of the world's population has an iodine deficiency, which is considered to be the leading cause of preventable mental retardation. For food sources along with recommendations for supplementation, see chapter 4.

• •

Eat a Good Breakfast

Many studies have shown that eating breakfast is important for controlling and maintaining weight over time, but *what* you eat for breakfast is also important. Foods that are low on the glycemic index and high in fiber—such as high-fiber cereals, fruit, and low-fat or nonfat dairy products—will keep you feeling full, so you'll be less likely to overeat at subsequent meals, and will keep your blood sugar level steady, which is the key to avoiding diabetes.

For some good breakfast options, see the cereals list (chapter 4), the recipes (chapter 10), and Dr. Steve's Probiotic Breakfast Special (chapter 5).

• •

And Don't Forget . . .

Keep on consuming all of the important antioxidant foods and nutrients already discussed in chapter 1.

Take Care of Your Oral Health

The bacteria in your mouth can affect your overall health as well as the health of your baby. Approximately 12.7 percent of U.S. births are preterm deliveries—a 36 percent increase in the last twenty-five years. Intrauterine infection is recognized as a main cause of preterm birth, late miscarriage, and stillbirth, and even though intrauterine infection has long been attributed to bacteria ascending into the uterus from the lower genital tract, recent studies indicate that such infections are also caused by bacteria in the mouth.

One study identified a diverse group of bacterial species colonizing the placenta of rats and found that the majority had originated in the oral cavity. These same bacteria are associated with adverse pregnancy outcomes in humans. The researchers therefore stated that "based on our findings, we postulate that periodontal therapies targeted at consistently reducing the total bacterial load in the mom's oral cavity may be effective in improving birth outcomes."

The human mouth harbors approximately seven hundred species of bacteria, and gingivitis (a mild form of periodontal disease) is a common problem during pregnancy. Having gingivitis means that you also have an increased chance of transmitting harmful bacteria to the placenta via your bloodstream. In fact, periodontal disease has been associated with poor fetal conditions, including preterm birth and low birth weight.

It is important that you get your mouth in tip-top shape before conception, if possible, because treatment of gum disease during pregnancy does not seem to significantly lower the chances of experiencing a preterm birth or having a low–birth weight baby.

To avoid this problem, have a dental exam and get your teeth cleaned before you become pregnant. Floss and brush with an electric toothbrush for two minutes twice a day. Eat lots of prebiotic foods, which promote the growth of probiotics (good bacteria) and prevent cavities and gum disease.

Some of the best prebiotic foods are blueberries, cranberries, tea (especially green), honey, grapes, raisins, dark chocolate, coffee, and barley coffee. The effect of diet on oral health is undeniable, and it has been shown that populations that consume high quantities of polyphenol-rich foods or beverages (such as Japanese tea drinkers) have a low incidence of cavities and better oral health overall.

Green tea and oolong tea have been shown to inhibit the cariogenic (cavity-causing) properties of certain oral bacteria, and cranberries (even more than tea) prevent cavities. My recommendation is to consume and swish around in your mouth coffee, tea, and cranberry juice. (If pure cranberry juice has too strong a taste for you, try diluting it with a bit of water.) Natural products derived from plants have provided numerous medicines, and the above data indicate that a natural approach can play a positive role in oral health. Using pure propolis toothpaste (available from http://www .holocuren.com) is also a good way to help prevent plaque formation. (Propolis is a substance in the buds of trees that bees collect and use to maintain their hives.)

Clean Up Your Microbiome

Microbiome refers to all of the bacteria in one's intestinal tract at all times. Everyone's microbiome is unique—like a fingerprint—and having a variety of good bacteria in your intestinal tract will help to ensure a healthy pregnancy.

Several recent studies have shown that the bacteria living in the intestinal tract significantly affect the way we metabolize calories. Animal studies have found that transferring the intestinal bacteria of an overweight animal into a thin animal will cause the thin animal to gain weight, and vice versa. We know that being overweight is a problem both before and during pregnancy, and we also know that whatever bacteria (good or bad) you have in your body will be passed along the food chain to your baby, both in utero and during a vaginal delivery.

Therefore, the goal should be to clean up your microbiome and fill it with as much good bacteria as possible so that you pass along a thin person's microbiome to your child. None of us can know exactly what bacteria have taken up residence in our intestinal tracts, but by eating a diet rich in SuperFoods, you will be increasing the chances that both you and your baby will have a thin person's microbiome.

And, Yes, If You Need to, Try to Lose Some Weight!

We've already discussed how being overweight or obese can affect fertility, but there are many other reasons why achieving a healthy weight before conception is so important. To determine your own health status in relation to weight, I urge all women planning to become pregnant to take two important measurements.

First, figure out your BMI, the measurement based on your weight in relation to your height. Go online to http://www.nhlbisupport.com/bmi/bmicalc.htm (or any of the several other BMI calculator sites online), type in your height and your weight, and the program will do the calculation for you. The ideal is a BMI above 18.5 and below 25. If it's too low, you may have fertility problems, and if it's too high, you may not only have trouble conceiving but also have other problems down the road during and after pregnancy; we'll discuss those in a minute. A BMI of 18.5 to less than 25 is considered normal; 25 to 30 is considered overweight; 30 to 35 is obese; and above 35 is morbidly obese. So if you can't get down to 25, at least aim to get below 30.

Second, calculate your waist-to-hip ratio. Possibly even more important than your BMI is *where* you carry your fat. If you tend to carry fat in your midsection rather than around your hips, you may be at greater risk for health issues, including insulin resistance (a condition in which you require more and more insulin to control your blood sugar), an elevated glucose level, an increase in inflammatory markers, hypertension, cardiovascular disorders, cataracts, age-related macular degeneration, and a number of other chronic diseases, and you may also be less fertile and have more problems during pregnancy.

It is estimated that 62 percent of women and 74 percent of men over the age of sixty-five carry excess weight in the abdomen, but the problem starts much earlier—often after your first pregnancy. Get control of your waist size now, and you'll be protecting your own health and the health of your child for years to come.

To determine your waist-to-hip ratio, measure your waist (about one inch above your belly button) and your hips (at their widest point). Divide your waist measurement by your hip measurement; that is your waist-to-hip ratio, which ideally is between 0.7 and 0.9.

• •

Nine Foods That Reduce Your Waistline

The following foods have been shown to reduce the waist-to-hip ratio:

1. Whole grains
2. Nonfat organic yogurt
3. Pumpkin
4. Tomatoes
5. Olive oil
6. Honey
7. Beans
8. Berries
9. Nuts and seeds

• •

With these two measurements in hand (and simply by looking in the mirror), you'll know whether you should be trying to lose some weight. There simply is no longer even a shadow of a doubt that being overweight or obese adversely affects fertility and pregnancy.

A study published in the *International Journal of Food Safety, Nutrition and Public Health* found that maternal obesity at conception affects gestational metabolic adjustments, the placenta, and fetal growth and development. Fetal development during the last half of pregnancy depends on maternal metabolic adjustments detected by placental hormones and the subsequent oxygen and nutrient supply, and if these are compromised through obesity issues, serious problems occur.

In another study, overweight women undergoing fertility treatment had double the rate of miscarriage compared to normal-weight women. More than one in three of the overweight or obese women in this study had a miscarriage, compared to one in five of the normal-weight women. The same study also showed a link between obesity and preeclampsia and/or premature delivery. My own conclusion from these findings is that all overweight women, whether or not they are undergoing fertility treatment, might be at increased risk for miscarriage as well as preeclampsia and premature delivery.

Obese women are also significantly more likely than normal-weight women to have children with congenital heart defects. And as the weight goes up, the risk continues to rise. Congenital heart defects are the most common type of congenital birth defect. In the United States, birth defects account for about 20 percent of infant deaths, and congenital heart defects account for about one-third of these deaths.

Women who are overweight before pregnancy also tend to be overweight during pregnancy, which predisposes them to gestational diabetes and having babies who are large for their gestational age (which predisposes the babies to childhood obesity). A review of more than sixteen thousand births showed that the odds of delivering an infant weighing more than 8.82 pounds were 70 percent higher for obese women.

When a group of 3,022 children born to 2,070 mothers were studied at six and seven years of age, 24 percent of those with obese mothers were obese themselves, whereas only 9 percent with normal-weight mothers were obese.

Overweight mothers are more likely to give birth to children who have weight-related health problems both in childhood and as adults. One of the known risk factors for childhood obesity is a family history of obesity. Compared to normal-weight children, obese children have been found to have a higher rate of dying by age sixty.

One large review study that looked at seventy-four thousand births found that the BMI of pregnant women increased between 1990 and 2005, and so did the ponderal index, a measurement of newborn body fat. A higher ponderal index means that a newborn's body has a higher percentage of fat, which in turn suggests that the risk for adult obesity and heart disease actually began before birth. At the present time, almost two-thirds of U.S. adults age twenty and older are either overweight or obese. The statistics for U.S. children are eye-opening: 11 percent of kids ages two to five, 15 percent of those ages six to eleven, and 18 percent of those ages twelve to nineteen are overweight or obese.

One study looked specifically at mothers and daughters and found that average-height women who weighed 150 pounds before pregnancy were twice as likely as those who weighed 125 pounds to have daughters who were obese at age eighteen.

A study of 3,022 children found that if a woman was overweight before she became pregnant, her child was as much as three times more likely to be overweight by age seven than a child whose mom was not overweight. In addition, the risk that a child would be overweight at a young age increased with the degree of the mother's obesity.

Rat studies have shown that babies born to obese mothers have too much insulin and genetic changes that put them at risk for fatty liver disease, which is now also being seen in human children.

Your weight doesn't only affect your child's health during gestation and after birth, it also affects your own. Obese women have an increased risk of a number of pregnancy complications, including gestational diabetes, hypertensive disorders, thromboembolic disease (such as blood clots in the legs or the lungs), and requiring a cesarean section.

A study that looked at 649 women, of whom almost half were overweight at the beginning of pregnancy, found that the overweight women were nearly ten times as likely to suffer from chest infections and more than twice as likely to have headaches and heartburn than the women who were normal weight. Finally, it is becoming increasingly clear that maintaining a healthy weight at midlife is directly related to enjoying a healthy longevity.

A subanalysis of the Nurses' Health Study evaluated self-reported weight at age eighteen and at midlife (mean age of fifty) in relation to health status, physical limitations, and cognitive status among participants who survived until at least the age of seventy. The women with a BMI of 25 at age eighteen were 33 percent less likely to be healthy after age seventy than the women with BMIs of 18.5 to 22.9 at age eighteen.

In addition, the women who were lean at age eighteen but who had gained more than twenty-two pounds by the beginning of the study were almost 60 percent less likely to be healthy than those who had maintained a stable weight until midlife. For every two pounds in weight gain since age eighteen, the odds of healthy survival fell by 5 percent.

The point here is not to scare you but to make it clear that if you do need to lose weight, the time to start is now, and that every single pound counts. Whatever you can do is better than doing nothing. You'll be increasing the chances that you and your baby will enjoy long and healthy lives.

• •

Dads Are Not Off the Hook

Recent investigations have shown that childhood weight gain correlates with paternal as well as maternal weight, and a 2010 study found that having two obese parents increased a child's risk of becoming obese twelvefold compared to the children with two healthy-weight parents. Parents play a major role in the increasing incidence of childhood obesity.

• •

The Good News

The good news is that once you start to eat the SuperFoods and the nutrients I recommend, you will begin to lose weight without having to think much about it. You'll feel full, you won't feel deprived, and you'll have more energy, so you'll also be more likely to get moving, which will help you to lose weight and keep it off.

• •

What Does a Portion Look Like?

The following are portion sizes according to the USDA:

Vegetables, chopped, ½ cup: ½ baseball

Raw leafy vegetables, 1 cup: 1 baseball or a fist

Fresh fruit, 1 medium: 1 baseball

Dried fruit, ¼ cup: 1 golf ball

Pasta, rice, or cereal, cooked, ½ cup: ½ baseball

Cereal, ready to eat, 1 ounce: can vary from ¼ cup (1 golf ball) to 1¼ cups (1 baseball + 1 golf ball)—read the label

Meat, or seafood, boneless, cooked, 3 ounces: a deck of cards

Beans, cooked, ½ cup: ½ baseball

Nuts, ⅓ cup: a level handful

Cheese, 1½ ounces (2 ounces, if processed): 1 ounce looks like 4 dice

• •

Here are a few tips for healthy weight control:

- Eat three healthy meals a day plus one midmorning and one midafternoon snack. Avoid skipping meals or saving up calories for one really big meal.
- Use smaller plates so that your portions will look bigger.
- Read food labels to learn what a "portion size" really is. Most of us underestimate the amount we're actually eating.
- Keep a food diary and write down all the calories you consume for five to seven days. This is a good way to get a picture of how much you're really eating.
- Always snack on whole foods, such as apples, pears, bananas, carrots, or celery with natural peanut butter. Avoid processed-food snacks. For a treat, try healthy chips such as those listed in chapter 11.
- Limit treats to 100 calories a day.
- Eat slowly. It takes about twenty minutes for the satiety nerves in your stomach to register fullness and send a message to the satiety center in your brain to "Stop eating! You are full."
- Eat more nonfat (preferably organic) dairy. Multiple studies have shown that increased consumption of dairy plays

a role in controlling weight and body composition, and environmental toxins are stored mainly in fat. Therefore, organic is best, but even if it's not organic, it should ideally be nonfat.

- When you go to the market, shop like a hunter-gatherer or a farmer. Avoid processed foods and buy more whole foods.
- Fill up on fiber for fewer calories.
- Limit sodium consumption to 1,500 milligrams a day by avoiding processed foods and the salt shaker. Spice up your food instead.
- Avoid sodas and other sugar-sweetened drinks. Try sipping water or tea with your meal instead. If you want a diet soda once in a while, you'll be better off with a clear soda rather than a cola, because colas leach calcium out of your bones. See chapter 11 for my two favorite "treat" sodas.
- Tune up your intestinal microbiome (discussed above) for better food processing.
- Don't eat in front of the television.
- Eat with family and friends.
- Limit restaurant meals to three or fewer a week. And when you do eat out, share an entrée, ask for salad dressing on the side, and have a bowl of berries for dessert. There is significant evidence that restaurant meals in general pack significantly more calories than most home-cooked meals. There are many reasons for this, including larger portion sizes, higher fat content (including saturated fats and trans fats), more sugar (particularly from soft drinks), and our tendency to indulge ourselves and make less healthy choices when we're eating out.
- Wear a pedometer and aim for ten thousand steps a day.
- Do strength-training exercises to maximize your lean body mass. Muscle burns calories even when you're sleeping!
- Get at least thirty minutes of physical activity six days a week.

- Reduce daily sitting time. It's bad for you and your waistline.
- When you're talking on the phone, stand up and walk around.
- Aim for seven to eight hours of sleep each night. See chapter 6 for an in-depth discussion of this important weight control strategy.

··

CONSUMER ALERT

Here are a couple of websites to visit to find a good pedometer:
http://www.pedometersusa.com/walkingpedometers
http://www.fitbit.com/pedometers
http://www.walkfithealth.com/

··

4

The Prepregnancy Nutrition Program: What, How Much, How Often

You now know which nutrients will help you get pregnant, but you still need to become aware of which foods contain the most of each nutrient, how much of each one you should be eating, how often, and whether supplementation will be useful.

This chapter contains the answers to all of those questions. It provides the quantities I recommend for each nutrient and how much each food will provide. In every case, the foods are listed in order of those that provide the most to those that provide the least. Even though all of these foods are health promoting, do be aware that eating too much of any food or taking in more calories than you expend will cause you to gain weight. So please be mindful of not overeating, and watch your weight.

You'll notice that many, if not most, of these foods appear on more than one list. That's because SuperFoods provide a multitude of nutritional and health benefits. So when you find those you enjoy the most, you'll no doubt also find that you're providing yourself with many different benefits at once.

The Twenty-Five SuperFoods and Their Sidekicks

The twenty-five SuperFoods and their sidekicks are all readily available and contain nutrients whose longevity-enhancing properties and contributions to optimal health have been substantiated by an ever-expanding body of scientific evidence.

Apples (and pears, bananas, and pineapple)	1 per day
Avocados (and asparagus and artichokes)	⅓ to ½ avocado or artichoke or 5 to 10 asparagus spears multiple times per week
Beans (pinto, kidney, navy, great northern, lima, garbanzo, and green beans; lentils; and sugar snap and green peas)	4 ½-cup servings per week
Blueberries (and purple or green grapes, cranberries, boysenberries, raspberries, goji berries, strawberries, currants, blackberries, cherries, and all other varieties of fresh, frozen, or freeze-dried berries)	1 cup daily
Broccoli (and Brussels sprouts, red and green cabbage, kale, turnips, cauliflower, rutabaga, kohlrabi, broccoflower, bok choy, collards, mustard greens, turnip greens, Swiss chard, arugula, watercress, daikon, wasabi, and liverwort)	½ to 1 cup most days
Chocolate, dark	No more than 100 calories per day; quantities will vary depending on the particular brand; read the nutrition panel on the label.

(continued)

Dried and freeze-dried fruits	2 heaping tbsps or 1 serving (according to the label) 3 or 4 times per week
Extra-virgin olive oil, first cold-pressed (and canola oil)	2 tbsps daily
Garlic	Multiple times per week
Honey	1 to 2 tsps daily
Kiwis (as well as strawberry guavas, pineapple guavas, and Brazilian or lemon guavas)	Multiple times per week
Oats (and oat bran, wheat germ, ground flaxseed meal, brown rice, wild rice, barley, wheat, buckwheat, rye, millet, bulgur wheat, amaranth, quinoa, triticale, kamut, yellow corn, spelt, and couscous)	Minimum of 10 g whole-grain fiber per day
Onions (and chives, scallions, shallots, and leeks)	⅛ to ½ cup most days
Oranges (and tangerines, tangelos, lemons, limes, white and pink grapefruit, and kumquats	Daily
Pomegranates or pure pomegranate juice (and plums, peaches, and nectarines)	Multiple times per week (if using juice, 4 to 8 ounces, with meals)
Pumpkin (and carrots; butternut squash; sweet potatoes; orange, red, yellow, and green bell peppers; mangoes; and apricots)	½ to 1 cup 5 to 7 times per week
Soy (tofu, soy milk, soy yogurt, soy nuts, edamame, tempeh, and miso)	10 to 15 grams of soy protein per day (quantity to be determined by the grams of protein in the product)
Spices (cinnamon, turmeric, oregano, peppercorns, and many other herbs and spices	As much as you want daily
Spinach (and kale, collard greens, Swiss chard, arugula, mustard greens, turnip greens, bok choy, romaine lettuce, and seaweed	1 cup steamed or 2 cups raw most days
Tea (green, black, oolong, white, and rooibos)	At least 1 to 4 cups per day
Tomatoes (and pink grapefruit, watermelon, eggplant, Japanese persimmons, red-fleshed papayas, and strawberry guava)	Multiple times per week

Turkey breast, skinless (and skinless chicken breast)	3 to 4 oz 3 or 4 times per week
Walnuts (and almonds, pistachios, sesame seeds, peanuts, pumpkin seeds, sunflower seeds, chia seeds, macadamia nuts, pecans, hazelnuts, pine nuts, and cashews)	1 handful 5 times per week
Wild salmon (and Alaskan or northern halibut, canned chunk light or albacore tuna, mackerel, sardines, herring, trout—farmed or wild—oysters, and clams—farmed or wild—crab, mussels, and lobster)	3 to 4 oz up to 4 times per week
Yogurt, nonfat, organic (and kefir, Greek yogurt, soy yogurt, DanActive Immunity, and nonfat organic milk)	1 to 2 cups most days

Seven Protective SuperFoods

The following are seven of the twenty-five SuperFoods that have been shown to be most effective for protecting your body against the detrimental effects of environmental pollutants.

Soy products	Aim for 10–15 grams of soy protein per day from whole-food sources.
Edamame (1 cup)	23 g protein
Tofu (4 oz)	18–20 g protein
Tempeh (½ cup)	16–19 g protein
Soy nuts (⅓ cup)	12 g protein
Soy milk (1 cup)	7–11 g protein
Soy yogurt (6 oz)	7 g protein
Miso (2 tbs)	4 g protein
Apples (and pears, bananas, and pineapple)	1 per day
Tea (green, black, oolong, white, and rooibos)	1–4 cups per day
Onions (and chives, scallions, shallots, and leeks)	⅛ to ½ cup most days
Garlic	Multiple times per week

(*continued*)

Broccoli (and Brussels sprouts, red and green cabbage, kale, turnips, cauliflower, rutabaga, kohlrabi, broccoflower, bok choy, collards, mustard greens, turnip greens, Swiss chard, arugula, watercress, daikon, wasabi, and liverwort)	½ to 1 cup most days
Spices	As much as you like, as often as you like

Sources of Vitamin C

The Recommended Daily Allowance (RDA) for vitamin C for males fourteen to eighteen is 75 milligrams per day; for females fourteen to eighteen, it's 65 milligrams. For men nineteen and older, the RDA is 90 milligrams per day, and for women nineteen and older, it's 75 milligrams. For men nineteen and older who smoke, the RDA is 125 milligrams per day, and for women nineteen and older who smoke, it's 110 milligrams. (But, of course, you shouldn't be smoking or exposing yourself to cigarette smoke in the first place.)

The RDA of vitamin C for pregnant women eighteen and younger is 80 milligrams per day; for pregnant women nineteen and older, it's 85 milligrams. For breast-feeding women eighteen and younger, the RDA is 115 milligrams; for breast-feeding women nineteen and older, it's 120 milligrams per day. Some authorities recommend that an ideal maintenance protocol for protection from environmental toxins consists of 3,000 to 12,000 milligrams of vitamin C per day, but the Institute of Medicine states the tolerable upper limit to be 2,000 milligrams per day.

My own recommendation is to consume as much vitamin C as possible from food on a daily basis and to take 500 milligram supplements two or three times a day. These supplements should preferably include polyphenols such as rutin, hesperidin, and quercietin (rosehips).

Yellow bell pepper (1 large)	341 mg
Red bell pepper (1 large)	312 mg
Guava (1)	165 mg
Green bell pepper (1 large)	132 mg
Orange juice, fresh (1 cup)	124 mg
Orange juice, from concentrate (1 cup)	97 mg
Brussels sprouts (1 cup)	97 mg
Strawberries (1 cup sliced)	97 mg
Papaya (½ medium)	85 mg
Orange, navel (1 fruit)	83 mg
Broccoli, fresh (1 cup chopped)	79 mg
Cantaloupe (1 cup chopped)	75 mg
Kiwi (1 medium)	57 mg

Sources of Lycopene

Aim for a total of 22 milligrams of lycopene a day.

Tomato sauce, canned (1 cup)	37 mg
R. W. Knudsen Very Veggie Low Sodium Vegetable Cocktail, from concentrate (1 cup)	22 mg
Tomato juice (1 cup)	22 mg
Watermelon (1 wedge)	13 mg
Stewed tomatoes, canned (1 cup)	10.3 mg
Tomato paste (1 tbsp)	4.6 mg
Ketchup (1 tbsp)	2.9 mg
Pink grapefruit (½)	1.8 mg

Sources of Vitamin B_{12}

The Recommended Daily Allowance (RDA) for vitamin B_{12} for males and females fourteen and older is 2.4 micrograms per day.

I'd suggest that men aim for 4 micrograms of vitamin B_{12} a day from food and 100 to 1,000 micrograms a day from supplements. The RDA of vitamin B_{12} for pregnant women of all ages is

2.6 micrograms per day, and for breast-feeding women it's 2.8 micrograms per day. Pregnant and breast-feeding women should aim for 100 to 300 micrograms per day from supplements.

Clams (3 oz)	84 mcg
Mussels (3 oz)	20 mcg
Crab (3 oz)	9 mcg
Sardines (3 oz)	6 mcg
Salmon (3 oz)	2.4 mcg
Beef, grass-fed (3 oz)	2.1 mcg
Nonfat yogurt (1 cup)	1.4 mcg
Egg (1 large)	0.4 mcg

Sources of Vitamin E

The Recommended Daily Allowance (RDA) for vitamin E for males and females fourteen and older is 15 milligrams per day.

I suggest that men should aim for at least 16 milligrams of vitamin E per day to increase fertility. For pregnant women of all ages, the RDA for vitamin E is 15 milligrams, and for all women who are breast-feeding, it's 19 milligrams.

Wheat germ oil (2 tbsps)	41 mg
Canola oil (2 tbsps)	13.6 mg
Peanut oil (2 tbsps)	9.2 mg
Almonds, raw (1 oz)	7.7 mg
Sunflower seeds, hulled and dry-roasted (½ cup)	6.8 mg
Wheat germ, raw (2 tbsps)	5 mg
Hazelnuts (1 oz)	4.3 mg
Orange bell pepper (1 medium)	4.3 mg
Extra-virgin olive oil (2 tbsps)	4 mg
Peanut butter (2 tbsps)	3.2 mg
Blueberries (1 cup)	2.8 mg
Soybean oil (2 tbsps)	2.6 mg

Sources of Zinc

The Recommended Daily Allowance (RDA) for zinc for males fourteen and older is 11 milligrams per day, and for females it's 9 milligrams. I suggest that males should aim for 11 milligrams per day from food to improve fertility.

The RDA for women nineteen and older is 8 milligrams per day. For pregnant women eighteen and younger, it's 12 milligrams, and for those nineteen and older, it's 11 milligrams. For breast-feeding women eighteen and younger, the RDA is 13 milligrams, and for those nineteen and older, it's 12 milligrams.

Oysters (6 medium)	43 mg
Beef, grass-fed (4 oz)	6.3 mg
Crab, Dungeness (3 oz)	4.6 mg
Turkey, dark meat (3 oz)	3.6 mg
Sesame seeds (¼ cup)	2.8 mg
Pumpkin seeds (¼ cup)	2.6 mg
Chicken, dark meat (3 oz)	2.4 mg
Nonfat yogurt (1 cup)	2.2 mg
Chickpeas (½ cup)	1.3 mg
Almonds (1 oz)	1 mg
Milk (1 cup)	1 mg

Sources of Selenium

The Recommended Daily Allowance (RDA) for selenium for males and females fourteen years and older is 55 micrograms per day. The RDA for pregnant women of all ages is 60 micrograms per day; for breast-feeding women, it's 70 micrograms. I suggest that men and women of all ages aim for 70 to 100 micrograms daily from food, and that the maximum supplemental dose of selenium for everyone not exceed 70 micrograms per day.

Pacific oysters (3 oz)	131 mcg
Brazil nut (1)	68–91 mcg

Oysters, farmed (3 oz)	54 mcg
Crab (3 oz)	40 mcg
Halibut (3 oz)	40 mcg
Salmon (3 oz)	40 mcg
Shiitake mushrooms (8 oz)	37 mcg
Shrimp (3 oz)	34 mcg
Turkey breast (3 oz)	33 mcg
Sunflower seeds (¼ cup)	21 mcg
Brown rice (1 cup cooked)	19 mcg
Egg (1)	14 mcg
Walnuts (1 oz)	5 mcg

Sources of Omega-3 EPA and DHA

For omega-3s in the form of EPA and DHA (as well as DPA, another omega-3 fat found in fish), the total Adequate Intake (AI) recommended by the Institute of Medicine for males fourteen to eighteen is 125 milligrams per day; for females fourteen to eighteen, it's 85 milligrams per day. For men nineteen and older, the AI is 160 milligrams per day; for women nineteen and older, it's 90 milligrams. The AI for pregnant females fourteen to eighteen is 110 milligrams per day, and for pregnant women nineteen to fifty, it's 115 milligrams. For lactating females fourteen to eighteen, the AI is 140 milligrams per day, and for lactating women nineteen through fifty, it's 145 milligrams.

This is an evolving field of nutrition, and my personal feeling is that males fourteen and older should aim for a total of 2 to 3 grams per day from fish sources plus supplements and that females fourteen and older should aim for a total of 1 to 2 grams per day.

For omega-3, I recommend three to four ounces of any of the following foods two to four times a week.

Food	Quantity	Total Omega-3	DHA	EPA
Alaskan king salmon	3.5 oz	3.3 g	0.9 g	1 g
Alaskan silver salmon	3.5 oz	1.3 g	0.6 g	0.4 g

(continued)

Food	Quantity	Total Omega-3	DHA	EPA
Alaskan sockeye salmon	3.5 oz	1.2 g	0.6 g	0.5 g
Alaskan halibut	3.5 oz	0.5 g	0.3 g	0.1 g
Pacific blue mussels	3 oz	0.9 g	0.5 g	0.3 g
Alaskan albacore tuna, BPA-free, canned in extra-virgin olive oil	3.75 oz	0.9 g	2 g	0.6 g
Alaskan sockeye salmon, BPA-free, canned with skin and bones	3.75 oz	1.5 g	0.8 g	0.5 g
Sardines	1 can	unknown	unknown	0.9 g
Rainbow trout, farmed	3 oz	0.6 g	0.4 g	0.1 g
Pacific oysters	3.5 oz	0.6 g	0.2 g	0.4 g
Arctic char	3 oz	0.6 g	0.5 g	0.1 g
Atlantic herring	3 oz	1.7 g	0.7 g	0.9 g
Pacific herring	3 oz	1.8 g	0.7 g	1 g

The first seven food entries are from Vital Choice, http://www.vitalchoice.com.

Sources of CoQ_{10}

There is no specific recommended daily allowance for CoQ_{10}. I would simply recommend consuming as many of these foods as possible.

Herring, marinated (3 oz)	2.3 mg
Soybean oil (1 tbsp)	1.3 mg
Canola oil (1 tbsp)	1 mg
Rainbow trout (3 oz)	0.9 mg
Peanuts, roasted (1 oz)	0.8 mg
Sesame seeds (1 oz)	0.7 mg
Pistachios (1 oz)	0.6 mg
Broccoli (½ cup cooked and chopped)	0.5 mg
Cauliflower (½ cup cooked and chopped)	0.4 mg
Orange (1 medium)	0.3 mg

Sources of Vitamin D

The Recommended Daily Allowance (RDA) for vitamin D for males fourteen to seventy years of age is 600 international units (IU) per day; for men over seventy it is 800 IU per day. The RDA for females fourteen to seventy years old is 600 IU per day, and it remains the same for pregnant and lactating women.

Cod liver oil (1 tbsp)	1,360 IU
Wild Alaskan sockeye salmon (3.5 oz)	670 IU
Albacore tuna (3.5 oz)	540 IU
Wild Alaskan silver salmon (3.5 oz)	425 IU
Pink salmon, canned (3 oz)	360 IU
Sardines, canned (3 oz)	250 IU
Mackerel, canned (3 oz)	244 IU
Wild Alaskan king salmon (3.5 oz)	222 IU
White tuna, canned (3 oz)	200 IU
Shrimp (4 oz)	162 IU
Milk or soy milk, vitamin D–fortified (1 cup)	100 IU
Orange juice, vitamin D–fortified (1 cup)	100 IU
Cod (4 oz)	64 IU
Cereal, vitamin D–fortified (1 cup)	40 IU
Egg yolk (1)	20 IU

Dr. Steve's Favorite High-Fiber Foods

You can't beat the weight- and waist-control properties of fiber, not to mention its ability to help control inflammation and blood sugar, which in turn helps to lower your risk for cardiovascular disease and cancer. In addition, fiber is loaded with phytonutrients—that is, nutrients found only in plant foods—that play a major role in optimizing your health.

Cereals, Whole Grains, and Bread

Aim for at least 10 grams of whole-grain fiber as part of your daily total fiber intake. I recommend that men aim for 35 to 45 grams a day, and that women—unless they are concerned about low hormone levels (see chapter 3)—should try for 30 to 35 grams daily, which is a bit more than the Institute of Medicine's recommendation of 20 to 35 grams.

Julian Bakery Cinnamon Almond Raisin Bread (1 slice)	12 g
Kashi GOLEAN (1 cup)	10 g
Post Shredded Wheat & Bran (½ cup)	8 g
Nature's Path 3 Generations Organic Flax Plus Raisin (¾ cup)	8 g
De Cecco Penne Rigate Whole Wheat Pasta, no salt added (½ cup)	7 g
Nature's Path 3 Generations Organic Heritage Flakes (¾ cup)	7 g
Nature's Path 3 Generations Organic Flax Plus Pumpkin Raisin Crunch (¾ cup)	7 g
365 Organic Chia Seed (1 tbsp)	5 g
Bran for Life Bread (1 slice)	5 g
Bob's Red Mill Organic Whole Ground Flaxseed Meal (2 tbsps)	4 g

Fruits and Fruit Juice

Raspberries (1 cup)	8.4 g
Blackberries (1 cup)	7.6 g
Whole Foods Organic Dried Goji Berries (½ cup)	7 g
Apple, with skin (1 large)	5.7 g
Avocado (½ cup)	4.2 g
Townsend Farms Organic Antioxidant Blend (1 cup)	4 g
Pear, Bartlett (1 medium)	4 g
Dates, Neglet Noor, pitted (5 or 6)	3 g
Dried plums, Sunsweet Bite-size, pitted (7)	3 g
R. W. Knudsen Organic Prune Juice (1 cup)	3 g

Legumes

Whole Foods 365 Organic Black Beans, dry (¼ cup cooked)	12 g
Eden Organic Kidney Beans, no salt added (½ cup cooked)	10 g
Green peas (1 cup cooked)	8.8 g

Health Valley Organic No Salt Added Lentil Soup (1 cup)   8 g
Eden Organic Black Beans, no salt added (½ cup cooked)   6 g
Pinto beans (½ cup cooked)   0.4 g

Nuts

Pistachios (1 oz)   3 g
Almonds (1 oz)   3 g
Walnuts (7 whole nuts)   2 g

Vegetables

Collard greens (1 cup cooked and chopped)   5.3 g
Libby's 100% Canned Pumpkin (½ cup cooked)   5 g
Sweet potato (¾ cup cubed and cooked)   5 g
Broccoli (1 cup cooked and chopped)   4.7 g
Butternut squash (½ cup cubed and cooked)   3.5 g

Sources of Zeaxanthin

Aim for 2 to 4 milligrams of zeaxanthin per day from food.

Orange bell pepper (1 medium)   6.4 mg
Goji berries, dried (25–35)   1.45 mg
Yellow corn, canned (1 cup)   0.9 mg
Japanese persimmon (1)   0.8 mg
Yellow cornmeal, degermed (1 cup)   0.7 mg

Sources of Lutein

Aim for 12 milligrams of lutein per day from food.

Kale (1 cup chopped and cooked)   23.7 mg
Spinach (1 cup cooked)   20.4 mg

Collard greens (1 cup cooked and chopped)	14.6 mg
Turnip greens (1 cup cooked and chopped)	12.1 mg
Green peas (1 cup cooked)	4.2 mg
Broccoli (1 cup cooked and chopped)	2.4 mg

Sources of Thiamine

The Recommended Daily Allowance (RDA) for thiamine for females fourteen to eighteen is 1.0 milligrams; for women nineteen and older, it's 1.1 milligrams daily. For pregnant and breast-feeding women of all ages, the RDA is 1.4 milligrams, and there are no tolerable upper limit or toxicity issues. The RDA for males fourteen years and older is 1.2 milligrams per day.

Brown rice (¼ cup cooked)	0.19 mg
Lentils (¼ cup cooked)	0.17 mg
Orange (1 medium)	0.11 mg
Sunflower seeds (¼ cup)	0.8 mg
Green peas (1 cup cooked)	0.4 mg
Black beans (¼ cup cooked)	0.4 mg
Corn (1 cup cooked)	0.4 mg
Asparagus (1 cup cooked)	0.2 mg

Sources of Pantothenic Acid

The Adequate Intake of pantothenic acid for males and females fourteen years and older is 5 milligrams daily. For pregnant women of all ages, it is 6 milligrams per day, and for breast-feeding women, it is 7 milligrams per day.

Sunflower seeds (¼ cup)	2.4 mg
Cremini mushrooms (5 oz)	2.1 mg
Avocado (1)	1.68 mg
Corn (1 cup cooked)	1.4 mg
Nonfat yogurt (1 cup)	1.35 mg

Sweet potato (1 medium)	0.74 mg
Lentils (½ cup cooked)	0.64 mg
Egg (1 large)	0.61 mg
Strawberries (1 cup)	0.5 mg
Broccoli (1 cup cooked and chopped)	0.4 mg

Sources of Folate

The Recommended Daily Allowance (RDA) for folate for males and females fourteen and older is 400 micrograms daily. For pregnant women of all ages, the RDA is 600 micrograms a day from food; for breast-feeding women, it's 500 micrograms.

Lentils (1 cup cooked)	358 mcg
Pinto beans (1 cup cooked)	294 mcg
Garbanzo beans (1 cup cooked)	282 mcg
Spinach (1 cup cooked)	263 mcg
Black beans (1 cup cooked)	256 mcg
Navy beans (1 cup cooked)	255 mcg
Kidney beans (1 cup cooked)	230 mcg
Green soybeans (1 cup cooked)	200 mcg
Soy nuts (1 cup)	177 mcg
Collard greens (1 cup cooked)	177 mcg
Lima beans (1 cup cooked)	156 mcg
Romaine lettuce (1 cup shredded)	152 mcg
Orange juice, from concentrate (1 cup)	103 mcg
Broccoli (1 cup cooked and chopped)	103 mcg
Asparagus (4 spears)	89 mcg

Sources of Vitamin B_6

The Recommended Daily Allowance (RDA) for vitamin B_6 for males fourteen to fifty is 1.3 milligrams daily; for men fifty-one years and older, it's 1.7 milligrams daily. The RDA for females fourteen to eighteen is 1.2 milligrams daily. For women ages nineteen to fifty, it's 1.3 milligrams daily, and for women fifty-one and older, it is 1.5 milligrams daily.

The RDA for vitamin B_6 for pregnant women of all ages is 1.9 milligrams, and for breast-feeding women, it's 2 milligrams.

Tuna steak (4 oz)	1.2 mg
Chickpeas, canned (1 cup)	1.1 mg
Salmon (3.5 oz)	0.7 mg
Banana (1 medium)	0.68 mg
Chicken breast (3.5 oz)	0.6 mg
Turkey breast (3.5 oz)	0.5 mg
Spinach (1 cup cooked)	0.4 mg
Asparagus (1 cup cooked and chopped)	0.2 mg
Broccoli (1 cup cooked and chopped)	0.2 mg
Bulgur (1 cup cooked	0.2 mg
Onion (1 cup chopped)	0.2 mg
Winter squash (½ cup cubed and cooked)	0.2 mg
Hazelnuts, dry-roasted (1 oz)	0.18 mg
Raisins, seedless (½ cup)	0.1 mg

Sources of Biotin

The Adequate Intake (AI) of biotin for males and females ages fourteen to eighteen is 25 micrograms daily; for men and women nineteen and older, it's 30 micrograms daily.

The AI of biotin for pregnant women of all ages is 30 micrograms daily; for breast-feeding women, it's 35 micrograms.

Egg (1 large)	25 mcg
Wheat bran (1 oz)	14 mcg
Avocado (1)	6 mcg
Whole-wheat bread (1 slice)	6 mcg
Cauliflower (1 cup raw and chopped)	4 mcg
Salmon (3 oz)	4 mcg

Sources of Iodine

The Recommended Daily Allowance (RDA) for iodine for males and females fourteen years and older is 150 micrograms daily.

Although the following foods are good sources of iodine, experts maintain that even the fortification of food will not provide an adequate iodine intake for pregnant and breast-feeding women, so the recommendation is that any woman attempting to conceive should take 250 micrograms as an oral daily supplement. The RDA for iodine for pregnant women is 220 micrograms a day; for breast-feeding women, it's 290 micrograms.

Seaweed (1 oz)	415 or more mcg, depending on the type of seaweed
Cod (3 oz)	99 mcg
Salt, iodized (¼ teaspoon)	89 mcg
Baked potato, with skin (1 medium)	63 mcg
Milk (1 cup)	56 mcg
Shrimp (3 oz)	35 mcg
Navy beans (½ cup cooked)	35 mcg
Turkey breast (3 oz)	34 mcg
Hard-boiled egg (1 large)	29 mcg
Tuna, canned in oil (3 oz)	17 mcg

PART 2

While Baby Is in Your Belly

Congratulations! You're pregnant. If you've been following the advice I gave in part one, you're already well on your way to ensuring a healthy, happy outcome for both you and your baby. But even if you've just started reading this book, don't think you've missed the boat. Go back and read part one and start incorporating more of the SuperFoods I recommended into your diet. It's never too late to take control of your health, and everything you do at this point to increase your consumption of good carbohydrates and protein—as well as the vitamins, minerals, antioxidants, and phytonutrients you need to stay healthy—will work to guarantee your unborn baby's good health.

Chapter 5 is titled "The SuperFoods Way of Eating for Two." That's not the same thing as using your pregnancy as an excuse to eat more. In fact, as you'll see, eating too much is bad for both you and your baby. Many studies have shown that women who gain more than the recommended amount of weight when they're expecting are putting both themselves and their babies at risk for a lifetime of health problems, not the least of which is developing type 2 diabetes. Women who are overweight are most likely to give birth to children who become overweight, thereby passing along all of the health issues that go along with that problem. However, women who don't gain *enough* weight may also be restricting the healthy growth of their fetuses by "teaching" them to hold on to the nutrients they do receive, which can lead to weight problems later in life.

The correct way of "eating for two" is to consume the optimum variety of nutrients in the proper quantities. We'll talk about what those nutrients are and which foods, or combination of foods, are going to provide them. Getting enough protein, for example, has been shown to protect a woman's daughters from breast cancer.

I'll also explain what various vitamins and minerals do and how they work in synergy to protect fetal health and promote a healthy life for your child well into his or her adulthood.

Getting a good supply of probiotics and a variety of antioxidants in your system will ensure that you avoid inflammation and provide a healthy environment for your baby in utero. How life starts, even before birth, has a tremendous influence on how that life will progress for years to come. In terms of health and longevity, life starts at conception, and the foods you eat during pregnancy will actually affect how your children's genes are expressed (or not expressed), which means that your children may be either protected from or predisposed to a variety of chronic diseases throughout their lives.

Beyond the foods you eat, the environment in which you live and your lifestyle choices will also be determining factors in your future baby's life. So in chapter 6 we'll talk about where to find environmental pollutants and how to reduce their toxic effects as well as why it is so important to talk with your doctor about medications you may already be taking—and certainly to avoid the use of recreational drugs. The chemicals in a pregnant woman's urine have been shown to be present in the amniotic fluid, cord blood, and infant's first stool, which means that whatever is entering your system is also in the system of your unborn child. Various chemicals have been shown to affect fetal development as well as babies' neurological and motor development and even the reproductive systems of males.

You may be surprised to learn how ubiquitous many of these toxic substances are in the products we buy for the home—from food packaging to cleansers to beauty enhancers. But as you'll see, there are also relatively simple ways to avoid many of them and to minimize their effects.

We'll also talk about the importance of getting enough physical activity and enough sleep. Physical activity improves cardiovascular fitness and helps to control blood sugar, both of which are extremely important for the health of you and your baby. Sleep is invaluable for stress relief as well as for the proper regulation of blood sugar and blood pressure. Many studies have shown that sleep deprivation contributes to weight gain and elevated inflammation at the cellular level. So I'll offer a number of strategies to help you get a better night's sleep.

Finally, in chapter 7 I continue the specific dietary guidelines that began before you became pregnant so that you can continue to consume the proper quantities of the particular nutrients that will ensure health and longevity for both you and your baby.

5

The SuperFoods Way of Eating for Two

I n previous chapters we talked about why it is so important that you clean up your microbiome and maximize your intake of the foods that increase your ability to carry a healthy baby to term and to ensure your child's continued good health throughout his or her life. Now that you're actually pregnant, eating the right thing is even more important, because whatever you put into your body is also feeding your fetus.

Feed Your Baby As You Feed Yourself

There is incontrovertible and constantly growing evidence to show that the way a pregnant woman nourishes herself, in terms of both macronutrients (proteins, carbohydrates, and fats) and micronutrients (vitamins, minerals, and phytonutrients) will have a significant and lasting effect on her own health and on the short- and long-term health of her child.

For example, the offspring of rats fed a low-protein diet had a 38 percent reduction in a gene promoter known to prevent breast cancer, and human studies also show a correlation between a low-protein diet during pregnancy and the future rate of breast cancer in the children.

Although protein requirements don't change significantly during the first trimester, during the second and third trimesters the recommended protein intake is 71 grams per day for a pregnant woman, compared to 46 grams per day for a nonpregnant woman. But this is just one instance of the myriad ways in which simply eating certain foods can increase or decrease your future child's chances of living a long, healthy life. In chapter 7 you'll find a list of my favorite SuperFood protein sources for pregnant women.

Other nutrients that are key to optimum fetal development and reducing the risk of potential chronic disease down the road are the following:

- **Vitamin A.** This is essential for renal, pulmonary, and cardiovascular function as well as vision, regulation of gene expression, immunity, and red blood cell production. Preformed vitamin A comes from animal sources and is absorbed directly into the body as retinol. On food labels, animal sources of vitamin A are called palmitate. Organic soy milk contains up to 2 percent of the RDA for vitamin A as vitamin A palmitate. Plant sources are called provitamin-A and are converted by the body into retinol. Of the three kinds of provitamin-A, beta-carotene is the one converted most efficiently, followed by alpha-carotene and beta-cryptoxanthin. We convert beta-carotene into preformed vitamin A twice as efficiently as we do alpha-carotene or beta-cryptoxanthin. See chapter 7 for food sources of all types of vitamin A.
- **Vitamin B$_{12}$.** This is a key player in the production and metabolism of amino acids, including methionine, which has a significant role in the production of methyl donors.

A "methyl group" is a group of chemicals, and methyl donors, including folate, vitamin B_{12}, choline, and betaine, facilitate the transfer of a methyl group from one molecule to another in a process known as methylation. Many important metabolic events are made possible by the transfer of methyl groups from one chemical structure in the body to another. For example, many of our genes can be activated or deactivated by the transfer of methyl groups, and the process of methyl transfer or methylation (the process of methyl transfer) is used by genes and cells to communicate with one another. Abnormal methylation is almost universally found in cancer cells. Vitamin B_{12} is also important for energy production from fats and protein, the synthesis of hemoglobin, pancreatic function, and the prevention of neural tube defects. For a list of foods rich in vitamin B_{12}, see chapter 4.

- **Vitamin C.** This is the master antioxidant vitamin that protects the body from environmental toxins and plays a role in the regeneration of other antioxidants. It is necessary for optimum brain development, neurological function, collagen synthesis, and immune function, and most other antioxidants in our bodies function better in synergy with Vitamin C. Vitamin C plays a positive role in the body's phase 1 and phase 2 detoxification systems; increases liver glutathione levels and the glutathione antioxidant enzyme systems; protects the lungs from air pollution; decreases organophosphate toxin damage to heart, lung, and liver tissues; and ameliorates toxic metal damage from cadmium, arsenic, and lead. For a list of foods high in vitamin C, see chapter 4.

- **Vitamin D.** This is important for the overall health of both mother and child. In my practice I've tested the vitamin D levels in hundreds of people, and they vary tremendously. So in my experience, the only way to know whether you have an adequate amount of vitamin D is to be tested (see chapter 3). For a list of foods rich in vitamin D, see chapter 4.

- **Vitamin K.** This is called phylloquinone when it origi-nates from plant sources and menaquinone when it comes from animal sources or from the synthesis of bacteria in the colon (which is not as good a source of vitamin K as was originally thought). The vitamin K family is essential for normal blood clotting, cellular growth regulation, and cell signaling activities as well as for the prevention of osteoporosis, vascular calcification, and cardiovascular dis-ease. For a list of food sources of vitamin K, with proper quantities, see chapter 7.

- **Calcium.** A major structural element in bones and teeth, calcium is important for blood vessel dilation and con-striction, muscle contraction, nerve impulse transmission, hormone function (including insulin), and the optimum functioning of many of our body's proteins and enzymes. Studies have also shown an inverse relationship between, on the one hand, dairy intake in general and calcium intake specifically and, on the other hand, the incidence of insulin resistance syndrome and obesity. Yogurt, in addition to being a good source of calcium, may contain the prebiotic inulin as well as vitamin D, both of which help to increase the absorption of calcium. High blood pressure occurs in 10 percent of pregnancies, and calcium metabolism plays a role in regulating blood pressure. For a list of calcium-rich foods, see chapter 7.

- **Folate.** This is necessary for the regulation of homocysteine (an amino acid); the metabolism of nucleic acid (the build-ing blocks of DNA and RNA); for DNA methylation (which is important for cardiovascular health and cancer preven-tion); renal, pancreas, and brain cell function; and the pre-vention of neural tube defects. For a list of folate-rich foods, see chapter 4.

- **Iron.** This is important for cellular energy production; oxygen transport and short-term storage; energy metabolism; the immune system; renal, pancreas, and brain cell function; and DNA synthesis. The third trimester is when the mother transfers the most iron to the fetus, so this is a particularly important time to be sure you're getting enough iron. Iron from animal sources is much more easily absorbed from our gastrointestinal tract than iron from plant sources, so this is the time to eat healthy forms of meat. For a list of iron-rich foods, see chapter 7.

- **Magnesium.** This is essential for energy production from carbohydrates and fats; nucleic acid and protein synthesis; the structural integrity of the bones, cell membranes, and chromosomes; transport of nerve impulses; muscle contraction; normal heart rhythm; cell signaling; and blood sugar and blood pressure control. For a list of foods rich in magnesium, see chapter 7.

- **Zinc.** This is essential for renal, cardiovascular, pancreas, brain cell and neurological functions; cell signaling (important for hormone release and nerve impulses); the regulation of gene expression; and the immune system. For a list of foods rich in zinc, see chapter 4.

CONSIDER A CARNITINE SUPPLEMENT

At least one study has shown that a lack of iron can lead to a reduced level of carnitine, a vitamin-like nutrient that is essential for turning fat into energy. Restoring the plasma level of carnitine with supplementation during pregnancy may therefore prevent the development of gestational diabetes, especially in overweight women, by decreasing the elevated levels of free fatty acids. Aim for 500 milligrams once or twice daily. I like acetyl-L carnitine v-caps from NOW products (http://www.nowfoods.com).

Keep Eating All of the Antioxidant-Rich SuperFoods

There has been a rapid increase in the prevalence of allergies in the past few years, and this may be the result of environmental exposures (such as the toxins we've discussed) interacting with genetic susceptibilities and interfering with the maturation and normal functioning of the immune system. A woman's diet during pregnancy is one of the main factors that may influence specific immune maturation events, allergic sensitization, and the incidence of childhood allergies. A number of studies suggest correlations between the status of antioxidants such as vitamin C, vitamin E, some carotenoids, selenium, and antioxidant rich fruits, on the one hand, and the development of asthma and, to a much lesser extent, atopic dermatitis (a type of eczema) and other allergies, on the other hand. So a diet based on antioxidant SuperFoods (fruits, vegetables, legumes, nuts, whole grains, and cold-water fish such as wild Alaskan salmon and sardines) will help to protect your child from the likelihood of developing skin allergies, asthma, wheezing, and allergic rhinitis.

Get Control of Your Blood Sugar

Numerous studies show that a woman's diet and weight during pregnancy will affect not only her child's weight but also his or her risk for developing diabetes. In fact, regulating your blood sugar is probably the most important thing you can do to protect both your own health and the health of your child. Every cell in your body and your child's body will be affected in a positive or negative way by your blood sugar level.

A mother's weight and blood sugar status are directly related to her child's risk of also becoming obese and/or diabetic. The children of diabetic women are more likely than other children to develop type 2 diabetes as teens or young adults. A study done in 2008 showed that the odds of an adolescent's developing type 2 diabetes were two and a half times higher when maternal diabetes was diagnosed before rather than after the pregnancy. And in another study done the same year, the adult children of women who had had gestational diabetes were eight times more likely to become diabetic.

Studies have shown that the rate of childhood obesity rises in tandem with a pregnant woman's blood sugar level and that untreated gestational diabetes nearly doubles a child's risk of becoming obese by age seven. When gestational diabetes is treated, however, the child's risk of becoming obese is significantly reduced; in fact, the children of women who were treated for gestational diabetes had the same rate of becoming obese as those whose mothers had normal blood sugar. Diabetes, as we all know, is significantly related to being overweight. When your weight goes up, your ability to control your blood sugar goes down. And the rise in childhood obesity is directly related to the rise in type 2 diabetes in children.

In addition, at least one study has shown that women with gestational diabetes have a greater risk of developing type 2 diabetes later in life, and the complications from type 2 diabetes can lead to a variety of other chronic diseases as well as to an increased risk of pancreatic cancer.

This is why it's so important to have your blood sugar checked before you become pregnant, get it under control, and keep it controlled during pregnancy.

Aside from making lifestyle changes (which we'll discuss in the next chapter), avoid processed and sugary foods and eat whole foods that are low on the glycemic index. For a complete list of foods with their glycemic index and glycemic load, go to http://www.mendosa.com/gilists.htm. Unlike the glycemic index, the glycemic load takes into account the amount of carbohydrates in a typical serving of each food, thereby providing a more accurate picture of the effect it will have on your blood sugar.

Also, increase your carotenoid intake. Diets high in carotenoids have been shown to decrease the rate of diabetes. For a list of carotenoid-rich foods, see chapters 4 and 7. And reduce your intake of fat—particularly saturated animal fat, especially from red and processed meats, and trans fat. Meat from wild game (including buffalo) and beef from 100 percent grass-fed cattle have never been shown to cause diabetes, because they are extremely lean, and whatever fat these meats do have is primarily in the form of plant sources of omega-3 fatty acids. An overall high-fat intake has been correlated with increased insulin resistance. However, mono- and polyunsaturated fats, such as first cold-pressed extra-virgin olive oil and walnuts, are much less likely to adversely affect insulin sensitivity.

In addition, there are specific SuperFoods that will help you get and keep control of your blood sugar, not only during pregnancy but also throughout your life. Beans, for example, are high in protein and good carbohydrates, which don't spike blood sugar. Honey helps your body to process blood glucose, and both nuts and peanut butter help to control blood sugar. In fact, one study has shown that women who consumed one ounce of nuts or two tablespoons of peanut butter five times a week had a 25 percent lower rate of developing diabetes.

Whole-grain fiber is also great for lowering insulin resistance, and one study found that people who ate more white bread than whole-grain breads tended to have the highest rate of type 2 diabetes. See chapter 4 for a list of my favorite high-fiber foods. Cinnamon performs many of the same functions as fiber (and it tastes good, too). Cinnamon slows gastric emptying (which makes you feel fuller longer), thereby helping to avoid the sudden spikes in blood sugar that can lead to insulin resistance. Cinnamon has also been shown to enhance insulin sensitivity, lower blood sugar, prevent glucose-induced tissue damage, and (in some studies) lower blood pressure. Sprinkle it on your whole-grain toast or cereal for added healthy flavor.

For a list of foods that help to control blood sugar, along with proper quantities, see chapter 7.

Other nutrients that will help you to fight diabetes (and many other chronic diseases) include calcium, magnesium, and zine (discussed above); chromium and potassium (see chapter 7); and vitamin E and omega-3 fatty acids (see chapter 4).

One interesting aspect of the relationship among fetal nutrition, overweight children, and the development of type 2 diabetes is that babies who receive suboptimal nutrition in utero and have low birth weight but are born into an environment where food is plentiful are those most at risk for developing diabetes. This is largely believed to result from what epigenetics pioneer Dr. David Barker called the "thrifty phenotype," which means that nutritional deprivation at critical stages of fetal development can lead to permanent changes in the structure and function of various organs.

In other words, the fetus "thinks" there's a famine and "learns" to store nutrients when they are available. Once that occurs, the child's body continues to function as though there were a food shortage even when food is plentiful, potentially leading to obesity and the diseases of obesity, including not only diabetes but also cardiovascular disease and some types of cancer.

Weight Is Still an Issue

We've talked about the importance of losing some weight, if necessary, before you become pregnant, but the amount of weight a woman gains *during* pregnancy also affects her future health and that of her child. Many women seem to think that being pregnant gives them a free pass to eat all of the foods they've been avoiding all their lives. They think, "Okay, I'm not going to look good anyway, so I might as well just indulge myself for once in my life," or they decide that since they're eating for two, they can eat twice as much. Although I can understand the temptation, nutritional science shows that it's not a good idea. And, in any case, you're not eating for two *adults*!

Postpregnancy obesity (and the attendant risk of developing type 2 diabetes) has been associated with the amount of weight a woman gains during pregnancy and how quickly she loses the weight after giving birth. In one study, women who lost their pregnancy weight within six months gained an average of only 5.3 pounds later in life; however, women who kept their pregnancy weight at six months postpartum were 18.3 pounds heavier later in life.

Other studies have shown that women who gained more weight than recommended during pregnancy by the Institute of Medicine guidelines had a higher rate of having children who became overweight—and almost half of American women exceed these recommendations. In one study, the children of these mothers displayed the following characteristics compared to the children of mothers who gained the recommended amount of weight:

- Two pounds heavier
- Larger waists by more than three-quarters of an inch
- 1 kilogram (2.2 pounds) more body fat
- Higher systolic blood pressure
- Higher levels of inflammatory markers by 15 percent
- Lower levels of HDL (good) cholesterol

In another study, the children of women who gained more weight than recommended were 48 percent more likely to be overweight than those who stayed within the guidelines.

In a study that looked specifically at mothers and daughters, the researchers found similar results. The daughters whose mothers gained fifteen to nineteen pounds during pregnancy had the lowest rates of obesity, whereas the daughters whose mothers gained more than forty pounds while pregnant were almost twice as likely to be obese at age eighteen and later in life.

This study also found that too *little* weight gain was linked to the daughters' rate of obesity. A pregnancy weight gain of less than ten pounds was correlated with a 1.5-fold increase in the odds of the daughter's being obese at eighteen and a 1.3-fold increase in her odds of being obese later in life.

The Institute of Medicine's recommended guidelines for weight gain during the course of a pregnancy, based on prepregnancy BMI, are shown in this table.

BMI	Recommended Total Weight Gain
Underweight: less than 18.5	28–40 lbs
Normal: 18.5 to 24.9	25–35 lbs
Overweight: 25 to 29.9	15–25 lbs
Obese: 30 or more	1–20 lbs

Provisional guidelines for women carrying twins are as follows:

Normal: 37 to 54 pounds

Overweight: 31 to 50 pounds

Obese: 25 to 42 pounds

Of course, you need to consult your own health-care provider to personalize this table for your individual situation.

In the *Expert Review of Obstetrics and Gynecology*, Dr. Raul Artal, chairman of the Department of Obstetrics, Gynecology and Women's Health at St. Louis University School of Medicine and a world authority on weight-gain and obesity in pregnancy, commented on the Institute of Medicine's most recent guidelines for weight gain during pregnancy: "Excessive gestational weight gain has been implicated in an intergenerational vicious cycle of obesity as overweight and obese mothers give birth to big daughters who are more likely to become obese themselves and deliver large infants."

As noted earlier, however, the rate of having overweight children was similar for women who gained insufficient weight (the thrifty phenotype hypothesis). In addition, a low maternal BMI has been correlated with intrauterine growth restriction, which also predisposes children to developing insulin resistance and/or type 2 diabetes later in life as much as high birth weight does. So the goal should be to keep your weight under control without starving either yourself or your baby.

Researchers have found that pregnant women on high-fat diets had a higher rate of having children who developed nonalcoholic fatty liver disease (NAFLD) in adulthood or earlier. NAFLD is a condition associated with obesity and caused by the buildup of fat in the liver. Until recently, NAFLD was considered rare and relatively harmless, but now it is one of the most common forms of liver disease that may progress to cirrhosis. The researchers concluded that "too much saturated fat in a mother's diet can affect the developing liver of a fetus, making it more susceptible to developing fatty liver disease later in life." Your daily saturated-fat consumption should not exceed 7 percent of your calories. Four sources of significant amounts of saturated fat are butter (63 percent), whole milk (57 percent), cheesecake (44 percent), and hamburger (36 percent).

Pile on the Probiotics and Prebiotics

In chapter 3 we talked about the importance of eating foods that promote good bacteria in the mouth, but having good bacteria throughout your gastrointestinal tract during pregnancy is especially important. One of the most important reasons is to avoid the inflammation and infections that are known to affect the healthy course of your pregnancy. Studies have shown that increasing your intake of probiotic dairy foods lowers overall inflammation in combination with providing a healthy vaginal microbiological environment that can reduce bacterial vaginosis, which has been correlated with preterm delivery. Preterm delivery has been shown to account for about 70 percent of infant mortalities and almost 50 percent of all postnatal neurological complications. In addition to probiotic dairy foods, adequate vitamin A intake (and to a lesser degree provitamin-A beta-carotene) before and during pregnancy may reduce the risk of bacterial vaginosis.

Other studies have shown that taking a probiotic supplement during pregnancy reduced women's rate of developing gestational diabetes. And some health-care professionals believe that probiotics can lower the risk of allergies and asthma in your child's future. There are no credible studies suggesting any increase in adverse pregnancy outcomes from taking probiotics, and they do not seem to pose any safety concerns for healthy women who are breast-feeding. My favorite probiotic supplement is Digestive Advantage by Schiff (http://www.DigestiveAdvantage.com).

Finally, we've already talked about the fact that the microbiome in thin people is different from that in overweight people, and now a study has shown that taking a probiotic supplement during the first trimester can help women to lose the weight gained during pregnancy more quickly. The researchers found that one year after childbirth, women who got probiotics along with dietary counseling (compared to those who received dietary counseling alone or neither counseling nor probiotics) had the lowest levels of central obesity (fat around the middle) as well as the lowest body fat percentage. Central obesity was found in 25 percent of the women who had received the probiotics along with dietary counseling and in 43 percent of those who had received counseling alone.

In no instance were the probiotics shown to have any negative effect on either mother or child. So this is certainly what I would call a win-win situation.

The most effective probiotic food source is yogurt. Look for nonfat, preferably organic yogurts that have the National Yogurt Association's live active cultures seal on the container. Here are some of my favorites:

- Cascade Fresh Fat-Free Yogurt
- Whole Foods 365 Organic Nonfat Yogurt
- Wallaby Organic Nonfat Yogurt

- Alta Dena Nonfat Yogurt
- Brown Cow All Natural Nonfat Yogurt
- Horizon Organic Fat-Free Yogurt
- Stonyfield Farm Organic Nonfat Yogurt
- Stonyfield Farm Organic Nonfat Greek Yogurt
- Yoplait 99 Percent Fat-Free Yogurt (It's not nonfat and not organic, but it has higher calcium and vitamin D_3 levels than most yogurts.)

CONSUMER ALERT

One of my favorite probiotic products is DanActive Immunity, a probiotic dairy drink made by Dannon. My only criticism is that it isn't organic. I drink it anyway, but we should all urge Dannon to make a nonfat organic version of this product.

Also remember to eat the prebiotic foods (foods that promote the growth of probiotics) mentioned in chapter 3: blueberries, cranberries, tea, honey, grapes, raisins, and dark chocolate. Green tea is particularly important. (For Dr. Steve's Green Tea recipe, see chapter 1.)

Stonyfield Farm yogurts contain inulin, a prebiotic nondigestible food ingredient. In addition, inulin-like fructans, types of fiber that also act as a prebiotic, are found in foods such as leeks, onions, garlic, asparagus, Jerusalem artichokes, and chicory.

• •

Dr. Steve's Probiotic Breakfast Special

For a quick and easy healthy breakfast, mix one cup of yogurt with fresh blueberries, sprinkle with some wheat germ, and drizzle with dark honey. Wash it down with green tea.

• •

A study published in the *American Journal of Clinical Nutrition* indicates that it would also be a good idea to add cocoa to your list of prebiotic foods. Cocoa contains flavonols (a type of polyphenol) that may improve intestinal health through prebiotic-like activity. In this study, the participants who consumed a high-flavonol cocoa drink daily for four weeks had a significantly increased growth of good bacteria compared to the participants who had a low-flavonol drink. The researchers also saw a reduction in C-reactive protein, a biomarker for inflammation (see chapter 3) and systolic blood pressure in the high-flavonol group. And there's no need to worry that the small amount of caffeine in cocoa will have any detrimental effect on your pregnancy.

• •

Dr. Steve's Hot Chocolate

In a mug, microwave one cup of vanilla soy milk and stir in one teaspoon of dark honey. Then add four to six tablespoons of cocoa powder (preferably Dagoba Organic Chocolate Cacao Powder or Rapunzel Organic Cocoa Powder—unsweetened and nonalkaline) or to taste. Stir to dissolve and drink immediately. Keep your spoon handy for scooping up any powder that doesn't dissolve completely. Enjoy!

• •

Revisit Folate

If you haven't already begun to increase your intake of folate, the food form of folic acid, *do it now*. See chapter 3 for the benefits and chapter 4 for the amounts you should be getting. There have been so many studies on the benefits of adequate folate and the risks of not getting enough that there should no longer be a question in anyone's mind about this issue. Folate deficiency early in pregnancy has been linked to less fetal growth in the first trimester, when essential organ development is completed, and hyperactivity in children.

Folate deficiency during pregnancy has also been linked to pre-term birth. In a 2007 study of 34,480 low-risk pregnancies, folate supplementation before conception was associated with a 50 to 70 percent reduction in the incidence of early spontaneous preterm birth, and the level of risk was inversely proportional to the duration of the preconception supplementation. So make sure that you have enough SuperFood sources of folate in your diet.

Take Pregnancy Vitamins

A study done in 2007 suggests that there is a substantial chemoprotective effect on children from exposure to multivitamins during gestation. For example, children born to women who supplemented their diets with folic acid–containing multivitamins had about a 30 percent lower rate of developing a pediatric brain tumor, a nearly 50 percent lower rate of having neuroblastoma, and about a 40 percent reduced rate of being diagnosed with acute lymphoblastic leukemia. Animal models clearly show a relationship between maternal methyl donor intake and the development of breast and colorectal cancer in adulthood.

In addition to folate, other methyl donors are riboflavin, vitamin B_6, vitamin B_{12}, certain amino acids, choline, and betaine. Recent scientific data suggest that women's intake of these nutrients during gestation may have an impact on the risk of cancer in the women's children later in life. It is likely that the very earliest period of embryonic development (the first days to the first few weeks) is the time when intervention (in this case, multivitamins) has the greatest potential effect, and the mother's vitamin B status during these periods is the most critical for maximizing the genetic health of the embryo.

The conclusion to be drawn is that a growing body of research shows that altering the maternal intake of methyl donors can lead to gene-specific changes in cancer-relevant genes and that these alterations may affect later (pediatric and adult) cancer risk in the children. So be sure to take a multivitamin—either one of those suggested in chapter 12 or one recommended by your doctor.

Get More Choline and Betaine in Your Body

Choline and betaine, along with vitamins B_6 and B_{12} and folate, play a major role in controlling the blood level of the amino acid homocysteine. A study published in the *American Journal of Clinical Nutrition* compared women in the highest versus the lowest groups for total homocysteine (tHcy) levels and found that compared to the women in the lowest group, the women in the highest group had a decreased fertility rate as well as a 32 percent increased rate of preeclampsia, a 38 percent increased rate of premature delivery, a 101 percent increased rate of delivering a low–birth weight infant, and higher rates of stillbirth, infants with neural tube defects, and infants with clubfoot. In addition, adults with an elevated tHcy level have an increased risk for heart attack, stroke, age-related macular degeneration, osteoporosis, depression, and Alzheimer's disease.

Several studies have shown that people with the highest dietary intake of choline and betaine have the lowest levels of various markers for inflammation, including homocysteine. Therefore, I recommend that everyone consume an abundance of the foods that contain these two nutrients, take a multivitamin supplement, and get a tHcy blood test. The ideal tHcy level is less than 11 micromoles per liter, borderline is 11 to 15 micromoles per liter, and a high risk is more than 15 micromoles per liter.

Having an adequate supply of choline is particularly critical for pregnant women because large amounts of it are delivered to the fetus across the placenta, and choline levels are six to seven times higher in the fetus than in the general adult population. Therefore, even though choline concentrations are higher in pregnant women than in nonpregnant women, the demand may exceed the supply.

Some research indicates that a high level of choline may reduce the rate of neural tube defects in the fetus. One study found that women in the lowest quartile for dietary choline intake had four times the rate of giving birth to a child with a neural tube defect than women who were in the highest quartile. Other studies have shown that the same is true for the rate of spina bifida and anencephaly (congenital absence of all or part of the brain). Animal studies have shown that increased maternal choline lowered the rate of breast cancer in the mother's offspring.

Furthermore, the offspring of rats given supplemental choline during the later stages of pregnancy, when the hippocampus (the part of the brain involved in memory formation, organization, storage, and appetite control) is formed, showed permanent modifications in brain structure that preserved memory function later in life. Although the same results have not yet been demonstrated in humans, it would seem to me that given the many benefits already associated with choline, this could be yet another.

Another study showed that higher plasma levels of betaine during the second half of pregnancy were associated with lower levels of homocysteine, and elevated homocysteine is a known risk factor for preeclampsia, premature birth, and very low birth weight.

For food sources of choline and betaine, with proper quantities, see chapter 7.

Some studies of pregnant mice have also shown that increased riboflavin (vitamin B_2) may boost the health effects of choline, and the researchers postulate that the same may be true for pregnant women. For good food sources of riboflavin, see chapter 7.

Get Your Omega-3: DHA and EPA

DHA and EPA, the two types of omega-3 fatty acids found mainly in fish, have been shown to have significant benefits for all pregnant women and their fetuses (and, of course, for men as well).

The recommendations for the consumption of EPA and DHA from oily fish vary from one source to another. The United Kingdom recommends one to two portions a week for pregnant women, with the upper limit imposed because of concern about contaminants in some species. However, all of the kinds of fish I recommend, with the exception of tuna, are safe for eating during pregnancy.

The European Food Safety Authority recommends 250 milligrams of EPA and DHA per day for healthy adults, with an additional 100 to 200 milligrams of DHA daily for pregnant women. And the Food and Agriculture Organization of the World Health Organization recommends that pregnant women consume a minimum of 300 milligrams of EPA plus DHA per day, of which 200 or more milligrams should be DHA.

The brain is approximately 60 percent fatty acids by weight, and DHA accounts for approximately one-third of that weight. It is estimated that most pregnant women are getting about 50 milligrams of DHA a day, but I believe that they should have an intake of approximately 500 milligrams of DHA and 500 milligrams of EPA daily to ensure healthy development of their babies' brains, eyes, and nervous systems (not to mention optimizing the mothers' health as well). I am not aware of any scientific studies showing any adverse consequences of taking this quantity.

In fact, many studies have correlated a diet rich in DHA during pregnancy and breast-feeding with healthy pregnancy, the mental and visual development of infants, and protection of the mothers from postpartum depression.

At least one study has shown that DHA levels in the umbilical cord were closely linked to visual acuity as well as cognitive and motor development in newborns. Although fish consumption remains controversial because of potential mercury exposure, the researchers concluded that the "benefits from eating fish with low contaminant levels and high n-3 [omega-3] contents, such as trout, sardines, and wild salmon, far outweigh potential risks, even during pregnancy."

CONSUMER ALERT

To get the latest information on fish that are high in mercury or other toxins, go to the Monterey Bay Aquarium website, http://www.mbayaq.org, and click on Seafood Watch.

You can also get information from the Environmental Protection Agency (http://www.epa.gov/mercury/fish .htm), the Environmental Defense Fund (http://www.edf .org), and the Marine Stewardship Council (http://www .msc.org).

Other studies have shown that women with higher intakes of fish during pregnancy have a small increase in gestational length; they also have children who score higher on tests of neural system development and have a lower rate of poor neurocognitive development and allergic and inflammatory disorders. One study showed that women with higher levels of DHA in their umbilical cord blood had a lower rate of having children with ADHD and overall behavioral difficulties at age ten. So it would seem that an adequate supply of essential fatty acids to the fetus is important for long-term behavioral outcomes in children.

A study done in 2011 showed that the children of women whose diets were higher in omega-3 during pregnancy had children with lower levels of adiposity (fat tissue) at the age of three, possibly because omega-3 affects the part of the brain that is responsible for appetite control. For good fish sources of DHA and EPA, see chapter 4.

Unless you have diabetes, another great way to get DHA from food is to have one DHA-enriched egg, such as Eggland's Best (http://www.eggland.com) on a daily basis. If you do have diabetes, you should consult your health-care provider about your egg consumption.

For information on fish oil supplements, see chapter 12.

Eat Your Omega-3 with Flavonoids

A recent study has shown that berries, which are rich in flavonoids, a type of antioxidant phytochemical, increase the bioavailability and therefore the blood and cellular levels of omega-3.

Break the Vicious Cycle with SuperFoods and SuperNutrients

Virtually all human traits and risks for disease are determined by a combination of genetics and environment. Furthermore, the study of epigenetics has shown that environment can affect gene expression, thus influencing the health of future generations in a multitude of ways. When you are pregnant, your body *is* your baby's environment, and what you put into your body therefore has a profound influence on your child's future risk for disease.

Recent studies have shown that the experiences of one's ancestors modify the regulatory factors affecting one's own gene expression in such a way that physiology and behavior are substantially influenced, and these transgenerational effects will persist if the factors that brought them about persist.

Nutrition is one of the most powerful tools we have for affecting gene expression. Nutrients, micronutrients, and phytochemicals can modify a number of processes associated with health and disease prevention, including hormonal balance, cell signaling, and carcinogen metabolism. Several of these processes are often modified simultaneously by bioactive food chemicals, and even minor dietary changes can profoundly influence the way genes are expressed. Therefore, the nutritional choices you make during pregnancy can stop or even reverse any negative genetic changes that resulted from the nutrition and lifestyle choices made by previous generations—or by the situations into which they were born.

A recently published study of 27,243 subjects in a variety of ethnic groups suggests that the risk for cardiovascular disease conferred by chromosomal abnormalities inherited from our parents may be favorably influenced by a diet that is high in fruits and vegetables. This confirms that we can suppress the expression of inherited "bad" genes and encourage the expression of genetic pathways that protect us from the number one cause of death in the United States.

In addition, a second study published in the journal *Free Radical Biology and Medicine* supports the idea that the environmental manipulation of cardiovascular risk factors can be achieved by consuming fruit and vegetables. In this study, blood flow was increased and systolic blood pressure was lowered by the consumption of either apples or spinach. I suggest you take a reading break right now, have an apple for a snack, and plan on including some spinach in your lunch or dinner. Both you and your unborn child will reap some health benefits from such an easy strategy!

All of this indicates that even though you can't pick your grandparents or your parents (although that might be nice), you can mitigate the effects they might have on your children and your children's children.

In the next chapter we'll look at the ways your environment and your lifestyle choices during pregnancy interact with your diet to affect your health and the health of your unborn child.

6

Optimize Your Lifestyle and Environment

Beyond the ways you nourish yourself and your baby, there are many other environmental and lifestyle changes you can make while pregnant that will have a significant effect on the lifetime health of both you and your child. These include avoiding products that contain known chemical toxins and avoiding environmental pollutants whenever possible.

If you already started making these changes before you got pregnant, that's great. Don't stop doing what you've been doing. And if you're just getting started, don't worry. It's never too late to start getting healthier, and if you're pregnant, there isn't any more important time to start. Go back and read chapter 2. Start putting what you learn there to work for you today, and keep moving forward.

Get Even More Serious about Going Green

We talked in chapter 2 about a variety of environmental toxins and why it would be a good idea to avoid as many of them as possible before getting pregnant, but now that you are pregnant, cleaning up your personal environment is more important than ever. The list of potentially dangerous chemicals in our earth, air, water, home, and food is long, and the list of their potentially dangerous effects is equally long.

The Toxic Substances Control Act, passed in 1976, gives the Environmental Protection Agency (EPA) the right to regulate new or existing chemicals. However, many of the already existing chemicals were grandfathered in, while others, including cosmetics and pesticides, were "generally excluded" from EPA regulation under the act. Since the passage of the act, the EPA has issued regulations to control only a few chemicals. And it would be impossible, in any case, for the agency to test every one of the thousands of new chemicals being produced every year.

The bodies of virtually all pregnant women in the United States carry multiple chemicals, including some that have been banned since the 1970s and others that are still being used in common household and personal care products. Among the most omnipresent of all types of chemicals are pesticides. According to the EPA, more than *eleven hundred million* pounds of pesticides are used in the United States every year, and a 2005 report issued by the CDC stated that detectable levels of fifty different pesticides were found in a representative sample of the U.S. population.

Many studies have shown that the chemicals found in a pregnant woman's urine are also present in the amniotic fluid, umbilical cord blood, and infant's first stool, which is composed of substances ingested while in utero. Clearly, then, these chemicals do cross the placenta, and in studies they have been correlated with increased rates of adverse health consequences such as preterm birth, birth defects, childhood morbidity, and adult disease and mortality.

Here's a list of the toxic substances that just one study found in pregnant women, along with the percentage of participants who were found to have each substance in their bodies:

Perchlorate (rocket fuel): 100 percent

BPA: 96 percent

Lead: 94 percent

Mercury: 89 percent

Cadmium (toxic heavy metal): 66 percent

DDT (banned pesticide): 62 percent

Endocrine Disruptors

Endocrine disruptors are chemicals found outside the body that when ingested can block, interfere with, or mimic normal hormone functioning. One of the times it is most dangerous to disrupt the normal functioning of the body's endocrine system is during pregnancy, when hormonal signaling is responsible for regulating fetal development.

Among the most ubiquitous and dangerous environmental endocrine disruptors are bisphenol (BPA), polychlorinated biphenyls (PCBs), and phthalates.

BPA

BPA is used in a variety of food packaging products, including storage and take-out containers, water bottles, and canned goods. Through leaching, BPA easily finds its way into the food chain and into our bodies. In addition to being used in food packaging, BPA is used to seal water pipelines, in dental sealants, in credit card and ATM receipts, and in medical equipment. In short, BPA is virtually impossible to avoid entirely.

Prenatal exposure to BPA has been shown to negatively affect brain development and increase susceptibility to cancer later in life.

A study done by the Kaiser Permanente Division of Research in Oakland, California, found that prenatal BPA exposure could adversely affect genital development in males and that the degree of the effect was proportional to the degree of exposure. Another study, published in *Molecular Endocrinology*, found that exposure in utero altered long-term hormone response and breast development in female mice, which could lead to an increased risk of breast cancer.

And still another study, conducted by researchers at the Harvard School of Public Health, found that increased levels of prenatal BPA exposure led to increases in behavioral problems, including depression and hyperactivity, in three-year-old children, and these effects were more pronounced in girls than in boys. The researchers concluded, "Gestational BPA exposures might affect endocrine or other neurotransmitter pathways and disrupt sexual differentiation of the brain, to alter behavior in a gender-dependent manner."

To avoid BPA exposure as much as possible, cut down on your consumption of canned foods or look for BPA-free cans (see the list in chapter 2). Buy liquids in glass rather than plastic bottles whenever possible.

CONSUMER ALERT

You can buy organic juices in glass bottles from the following:

- R. W. Knudsen (http://www.rwknudsenfamily.com)
- Langers Juices (http://langers.com)

For bottled water, Glaceau Smart Water (1-877-GLACEAU) comes in BPA-free, recyclable number 1 plastic bottles. It also has added calcium, magnesium, and potassium. This is good because in areas of the United States where the water is naturally high in minerals, the rates of cardiovascular disease are lower.

Store leftovers in glass containers and transfer store-bought foods from plastic to glass as soon as you get them home. Don't microwave in plastic, because the BPA is more likely to leach when the food is hot.

CONSUMER ALERT

Stay away from plastic containers marked with the recycling code number 3, 6, or 7 or the letters PC (for polycarbonate). Plastics with the recycling labels 1, 2, 4, or 5 on the bottom are better choices because they do not contain BPA.

REI (http://www.rei.com) makes a wide variety of BPA-free reusable water bottles. Anchor Hocking, Kinetic Go Green, and Klip It all make BPA-free food storage containers available from a variety of sources.

A rat study has shown that aside from avoiding the sources of BPA, you can cut down on the effects BPA might have on your unborn child by making sure that your diet is rich in folate, choline, and genistein, an antioxidant found in fava beans and soybeans. (For sources of folate and choline, see chapters 4 and 7, respectively.)

PCBs

PCBs are industrial chemicals that were used as coolants and insulating fluids for transformers and capacitors, as plasticizers in paints and cements, in flexible polyvinyl chloride (PVC) coatings of electrical wiring and electronic components, and for many other purposes. PCBs were banned in the United States in 1979 but persist in the environment to this day.

The EPA, the International Agency for Research on Cancer, the National Cancer Institute, the World Health Organization, and the

Agency for Toxic Substances and Disease Registry have all classified PCBs as probable human carcinogens. PCBs have also been implicated in a wide range of other health issues, including effects on the immune system, the reproductive system, the nervous system, and the endocrine system.

PCB exposure has been found to reduce the birth weight, conception rates, and live birth rates of monkeys, and these effects continued to be observed long after the dosing with PCBs had stopped.

In addition, the effects of PCBs on nervous system development have been studied in monkeys and other animal species. Newborn monkeys exposed to PCBs showed persistent and significant deficits in neurological development, including visual recognition, short-term memory, and learning. Human studies have suggested similar effects, including learning deficits and changes in activity. Proper development of the nervous system is critical for early learning and can have potentially significant implications for the health of individuals throughout their lifetimes.

One study followed eight hundred pairs of mothers and babies living near the toxin-contaminated harbor in New Bedford, Massachusetts, from 1993 to 1998. The researchers measured the levels of organochlorine in the umbilical cord serum at birth and then used the Conners Rating Scale for Teachers to assess ADHD-like behaviors when the children were eight years old. They found that the rate of these behaviors increased from 26 to 92 percent, depending on the type of organochlorines to which the mothers and babies had been exposed.

Other investigators have found developmental and cognitive disorders in the children of mothers who had eaten moderate to high amounts of contaminated fish during the six years preceding a pregnancy and during the pregnancy itself.

PCBs were correlated to earlier births and several developmental effects, including lower birth weight and smaller head circumference, all of which were still observed when the babies were five to seven months old. The neurobehavioral problems linked to PCBs included depressed responsiveness, impaired visual recognition, and poor short-term memory at seven months old.

At four years of age, the children still had deficits in weight gain, depressed responsiveness, and reduced visual recognition and memory. At eleven years old, they were three times as likely to have low verbal IQ scores, twice as likely to be at least two years behind in reading comprehension, and also more likely to have difficulty paying attention.

In addition, PCB exposure is known to suppress the immune system in both humans and animals, and immune suppression has been shown to be a risk factor for non-Hodgkin's lymphoma, so this may be a mechanism for PCB-induced cancers.

The most common source of PCB exposure in humans is through food. The toxins are stored in the fat of fish living in PCB-contaminated waters and in animals that drink the water or are exposed to PCBs in the soil or in their food (a good reason to stay away from any kind of high-fat animal products, from marbled meats to full-fat dairy products). One of the reasons it's a good idea to lose weight before but not during pregnancy is that we too store PCBs in fat, and when we mobilize fat during weight loss, the poisons are released into our bloodstream and are then more likely to be transferred to the fetus.

Both the EPA and the Wisconsin Department of Health Services suggest that the fish with the highest levels of PCB contamination are likely to be bottom-feeders and those at the top of the food chain. In general, that means eating smaller, younger fish. Small organisms absorb contaminants in the water, and these organisms are then eaten by small fish. Big fish eat the small fish, and the contaminants accumulate up the food chain, with those at the top containing the most contaminants.

In addition, because PCBs are stored in fat, it's better to eat smaller, leaner, shorter-lived fish (for example, herring and sardines), which often have very low to undetectable levels of PCBs.

For more tips on how to limit your PCB exposure, see chapter 2.

Phthalates

Phthalates are a group of chemicals used to make plastics more flexible and harder to break. They're used in hundreds of products, including vinyl flooring, adhesives, detergents, lubricating oils, automotive plastics, plastic raincoats, shower curtains, and personal care products such as soaps, deodorants, moisturizers, shampoos, hair sprays, and nail polish. In addition, they're in many PVC plastics used to make plastic bags, garden hoses (which makes me wonder about all the water I drank from our garden hose when I was growing up), inflatable toys, blood storage containers, medical tubing, and children's toys. Whereas BPA makes plastic hard, phthalates keep it soft. And they are powerful endocrine disruptors.

Over the past forty years, many articles in peer-reviewed scientific journals have linked phthalate exposure to serious health problems in children, including early puberty in girls and reduced testosterone levels, lowered sperm counts, and genital defects in boys.

In 2001 the European Union classified two phthalates prohibited in toys (DEHP and DBP) as category 2 substances, defined as chemicals "which should be regarded as if they impair fertility in humans" and "which should be regarded as if they cause developmental toxicity in humans." The most commonly used phthalate, DEHP, is known to have an antiandrogenic (antitestosterone) effect, an estrogenic effect, or both. There seems to be a relationship between DEHP exposure and the incidence of early pubertal onset of an abnormal enlargement of the breasts in a male.

Various studies have shown associations between maternal exposure to a range of persistent environmental contaminants, including PCBs and phthalates, during pregnancy and an increased risk of testicular dysgenesis syndrome, which includes one or both testicles undescended, abnormal placement of the opening through which urine and semen exit the penis, and an increased risk for testicular cancer. An article published in the *Oxford Journal* suggests that "poor semen quality, testis cancer, undescended testis and hypospadias are symptoms of one underlying entity, the testicular dysgenesis syndrome (TDS), which may be increasingly common due to adverse environmental influences."

One of the most discussed studies correlating maternal phthalate exposure to male genital abnormalities was published in 2005. In this study, Dr. Shanna Swan and her colleagues found that human phthalate exposure during pregnancy results in decreased anogenital distance (the distance between the anus and the genitalia) in baby boys. Boys born to mothers with the highest levels of phthalates were seven times more likely to have a shortened anogenital distance.

In addition to finding sex-related issues, research has shown phthalates to be correlated with altered neurological development and behavioral problems in children. One such study found that higher prenatal exposure to phthalates was connected with disruptive and other problem behaviors in children.

Phthalate metabolite levels were analyzed in the prenatal urine samples of a multiethnic group of 404 women who were pregnant for the first time, and 188 of them were then interviewed when their children were between the ages of four and nine. The women were not informed of their phthalate metabolite level, and the researchers were unaware of their exposures when testing the children. They found that the mothers with higher concentrations of phthalates consistently reported poorer behavior profiles in their children, particularly in terms of conduct and externalizing problems (that is, behaving aggressively toward others)—characteristics typically associated with oppositional defiant disorder, conduct disorder, and ADHD.

Another study looked at the urine concentration levels in children themselves (rather than in pregnant women) and also found a significant correlation between phthalate exposure and behaviors related to ADHD.

Finally, at least one study has shown a correlation between high phthalate levels and low birth weight in infants. And researchers at the University of Michigan School of Public Health found that women who deliver prematurely have an average of up to three times the phthalate level in their urine as women who carry to term.

The EPA says that food is probably the main source of contamination. DEHP is commonly used in shipping and storage containers and can leach into foods and liquids, particularly if the container is heated or scratched.

Phthalates are also in the artificial fragrances added to many personal care and cleaning products and can be absorbed through the skin or inhaled. Because phthalates are in so many products we use every day, people are commonly exposed to them, and most Americans tested by the CDC have metabolites of multiple phthalates in their urine. There are, however, several ways to cut down on your phthalate exposure without making yourself crazy. Here are a few tips from *The Daily Green* (http://www.thedailygreen.com /environmental-news/latest/phthalates-47020418):

- Read the ingredients. According to the organization Pollution in People, you can identify phthalates in some products by their chemical names or abbreviations:
  - DBP (di-n-butyl phthalate) and DEP (diethyl phthalate) are often found in personal care products, including nail polishes, deodorants, perfumes and colognes, aftershave lotions, shampoos, hair gels, and hand lotions.
  - DEHP (di-2-ethylhexyl phthalate) or Bis (2-ethylhexyl phthalate) is used in PVC plastics, including some medical devices.
  - BzBP (benzylbutyl phthalate) is used in some flooring, car products, and personal care products.
  - DMP (dimethyl phthalate) is used in insect repellent and some plastics (as well as rocket propellant).
- Be wary of the term *fragrance* (unless it is *natural fragrance*). This is used to denote a combination of compounds, possibly including phthalates, which are a subject of recent concern because of studies showing they can mimic certain hormones.

- Choose plastics with the recycling code 1, 2, 4, or 5. Recycling codes 3, 6, and 7 are more likely to contain BPA or phthalates.

For additional information on products that do or do not contain phthalates, check out these websites:

- http://lesstoxicguide.ca/index.asp?fetch=usage
  This is the Environmental Health Association of Nova Scotia's Guide to Less Toxic Products, which lists toxins found in cosmetics and personal care products and provides lists of best, good, and simply unscented products in a variety of categories.
- http://www.cosmeticsdatabase.com/index.php
  The Environmental Working Group lists its "cosmetics champions," including the ingredients found in products from more than three hundred companies.
- http://householdproducts.nlm.nih.gov/
  The U.S. Department of Health and Human Services Household Products database has information on a range of chemical products that are found in and around our homes.
- http://www.cdc.gov/biomonitoring/BzBP_Biomonitoring-Summary.html
  The CDC has a comprehensive summary of phthalates and other chemicals found in the environment.

• •

Manufacturers and Sellers of Phthalate-Free Products

OPI, a leading manufacturer of professional nail products worldwide, has removed the phthalate DBP from its products.

Burt's Bees (http://www.burtsbees.com) does not use any synthetic fragrances that contain phthalates.

Whole Foods' website states that it does not allow phthalates in any tier of its eco-scale rating system for cleaning products (http://www.wholefoodsmarket.com/eco-scale/unacceptable.php).

Many homecare items found in supermarkets now have "phthalate free" or "no phthalates" or "fragrance free" or "natural fragrance" stated on the packaging.

• •

Pesticides

In 2002 the EPA stated that eleven hundred million pounds of pesticides are used in the United States annually and that approximately 90 percent of U.S. households use them. The problem is that even though all pesticides must be registered with the EPA, the law does not require any original research into the potential human health effects from exposure. In chapter 2 we discussed what some of those health problems could be and provided a number of ways to avoid them. Here are a few more very good reasons to stay away from pesticides—particularly when you're pregnant.

According to the research, a mother's occupational exposure to pesticide use before and during pregnancy was correlated with an increased rate of acute lymphocytic leukemia, Wilms tumor (a type of kidney cancer occurring in children), and brain cancer in her children.

A 2010 study conducted in two low-income New York City neighborhoods, the South Bronx and Upper Manhattan, showed a clear correlation between exposure to the organophosphate pesticide chlorpyrifos (chlorp) and delayed mental and motor skill development in children. The research indicated that high chlorp exposure was associated with a 6.5-point decrease in the Psychomotor Development Index score and a 3.3-point decrease in the Mental Development Index score in three-year-olds. Furthermore, these correlations remained statistically significant and similar in magnitude after dilapidated housing and other neighborhood characteristics were accounted for. In other words, this is not an issue simply for people who live in low-income neighborhoods.

Also interesting is the fact that even though chlorp has been banned for virtually all home uses since 2000 and is allowed only for agricultural use, it was present in the urban areas used for this study. The researchers concluded that the chemicals probably drifted from fields to nearby yards and also traveled with wind and rain to areas hundreds of miles from where they were used. This is a perfect example of why we should "act locally and think globally," as environmentalists recommend.

Like other environmental toxins, pesticides have been associated with genital abnormalities in the sons of exposed women. In addition to causing testicular dysgenesis syndrome (see above), pesticides have also been shown to increase the rate of undescended testicles in the sons of women who had the highest levels in their breast milk and in the sons of women who worked in greenhouses where pesticides were used.

Given the persistence of pesticides in the environment, there is probably no way to escape exposure to them altogether. In fact, of the twelve most dangerous and persistent chemicals identified by the Stockholm Convention on Persistent Organic Pollutants in 2001, ten were pesticides. But we can still significantly limit the effects they might have on us by not bringing them into our homes or our yards. It's better for you, your children, and the family pets. So keep pesticides out of your yard and remove your shoes before entering your home.

In chapter 2 we suggested a variety of alternatives to pesticides in the garden. Here are a few more to consider:

- Greenscapes (http://greenscapes.org/Page-143.html) suggests, "Put up bird feeders and bat houses to attract natural predators of insects. Birds and bats in your yard will consume insects by the thousands and provide you with entertainment, too. Attracting birds and bats will not increase the likelihood of them moving into your attic or wall spaces." If bats aren't your thing, at least go for the birds!

- Put up a barn owl box in the yard. A barn owl family will eat approximately two thousand rodents a year. That's a lot better than putting out poison to kill them. We have barn owls, and they've produced at least two babies each year since we've put up the box. We don't have any rodents.
- Bring in praying mantises, ladybugs, lacewing insects, and chickens (if it's legal where you live). All of these will keep the"bad bug"population under control and fertilize your garden. Earthworms are also great natural fertilizers. And chickens, if you're allowed to keep them, eat horse fly larvae and eggs. We have several horses, dozens of free range chickens (they even nest in our yard), and we don't have any horseflies. Limit roosters, as they"crow"long before sunrise!
- Beyond Pesticides (http://www.beyondpesticides.org /alternatives/factsheets/index.htm) has fact sheets that help you to identify a wide range of garden pests and weeds and offers suggestions for getting rid of them without pesticides.
- Gardens Alive (http://www.gardensalive.com/article .asp?ai=170) publishes *Purdue University's Guide to Pesticide Alternatives*, which offers products that will take care of pests inside and outside your home without the use of pesticides.

In addition, store food in tightly closed glass containers, be sure to clean up food spills and crumbs, remove standing water from leaky faucets, keep outdoor plants, shrubs, and trees from touching the walls of your home, and seal any cracks or holes that would allow pests to get in from the outside.

* * *

Websites to Help You Go Green and Stay Sane

Here are a few more Internet resources you can use to detox your environment.

http://www.healthyindoorair.org
http://www.ecos.com
http://www.simplegreen.com
http://www.thegreenguide.com
http://www.versatilevinegar.org
http://www.armhammer.com
http://www.audubon.org
http://www.nwf.org
http://www.ewg.org
http://www.EverydayExposures.com (great for identifying the toxins that are present in your home)

And don't forget distilled white vinegar, a great nontoxic way to clean. It's a staple in my home.

• •

Talk to Your Doctor about Medications

If you've ever wondered why women are told to avoid taking medications while pregnant, what you've learned about how substances cross the placenta or pass from the mother's bloodstream to her fetus should have answered that question somewhat. In addition, you should know that much of the umbilical cord venous blood flow bypasses the liver (the primary detoxifying organ), so the fetus is generally exposed to high levels of unmetabolized (unprocessed) blood. Because the developing child's liver is still immature, it has relatively little drug-metabolizing capacity. That fact, combined with the fetus's limited capacity to excrete drugs, means that your unborn child will be exposed to high and prolonged levels of whatever drug you take.

Because pregnant women are excluded from most clinical trials and data from animal studies are not always predictive for humans, the effects on fetal development and birth defects caused by drugs are unknown for more than 90 percent of all drug treatments. Because so much is unknown, it seems only reasonable to err on the side of caution. And there are some drugs we do know to be harmful.

Drugs that are known to affect fetal growth and other long-term health problems include the following:

Alcohol

Nicotine

Heroin

Cocaine

Marijuana

Methadone

Methamphetamine

Opiates

Phencyclidine (PCP; angel dust)

Steroids

Immunosuppressive drugs

• •

The Dangers of Cocaine

Dopamine, norepinephrine, and serotonin are neurotransmitters sending signals to the brain that are important for regulating a wide range of behaviors, cognitive functions, and moods. Dopamine abnormalities appear to contribute to many neurological and psychiatric disorders, including schizophrenia, Parkinson's disease, ADHD, and drug addiction. Norepinephrine is involved in mediating attention, anxiety, arousal, feeding behaviors, learning, and memory. Serotonin modulates sleep, sexual urge, anxiety, appetite, temperature regulation, learning, memory, and mood. Studies of effects of prenatal cocaine exposure suggest that the drug can affect the formation and functioning of brain circuitry so that these transmitters are not functioning the way that they should, leading to poorer perceptual reasoning, impairments in procedural learning, increased behavior problems in school, and increased rates of oppositional defiant disorder and ADHD.

• •

You shouldn't be taking illegal recreational drugs in any case, but you may be taking steroids or immunosuppressive drugs for legitimate medical conditions. If so, you should always talk to your doctor about what to do about any drugs you take (including over-the-counter drugs) while you're pregnant.

STAY AWAY FROM SPEED

Amphetamine or methamphetamine, commonly known as speed, has been shown to increase premature delivery, placental abruption, cardiac defects, fetal distress, and fetal growth impairment. In one small retrospective study, significant deficits in visual perception and visual control of movements (particularly eye movement), attention, and memory have been observed and linked to smaller volumes of certain parts of the brain. In animal studies, prenatal exposure to speed at high doses has induced prominent birth defects, selective effects on spatial learning and memory, and both transient and permanent effects in stress hormones and other brain chemicals.

One preliminary study has shown that first-trimester fetal exposure to the amphetamine known as Ecstasy increased the rates of cardiovascular and musculoskeletal abnormalities.

Drugs Associated with a Variety of Negative Outcomes

- **Folic acid antagonists.** These include a range of drugs used to treat epilepsy, mood disorders, hypertension, and infections. We already know how important it is to have an adequate supply of folate during pregnancy, so drugs that interrupt or limit the actions of folate are naturally dangerous to take during pregnancy. They have been correlated with increased rates of preeclampsia, placental abruption, fetal growth restriction, fetal death, neural tube defects, congenital heart malformations, cleft lip and palate, and urinary tract defects.

- **Selective serotonin reuptake inhibitors (SSRIs).** This class of drugs is widely used to treat depression. In a study using the Danish nationwide registry, the prevalence of major congenital malformations was similar for both the exposed and the nonexposed infants, but the prevalence of septal membrane heart defects was twice as high among exposed infants, and the rate among infants of women who took more than one type of SSRI was four times higher than among infants who were not exposed. The researchers remarked that the absolute risk for septal defects is small and that they can be minor and self-resolving. Depression affects up to 20 percent of pregnant women, and the benefits of pharmacological treatment must be balanced against the risks associated with fetal exposure. That said, however, a recent study has suggested that the children of women who took SSRIs during pregnancy might be at increased risk for drug abuse in the future.

Recent recommendations of the American Congress (formerly College) of Obstetrics and Gynecology (ACOG) state that the maternal benefits of SSRI use during pregnancy can outweigh the risks of prenatal SSRI exposure. A joint workshop of the American Psychiatric Association and ACOG reviewed the literature and found that in some studies, depression itself was correlated with higher rates of miscarriage, preterm birth, fetal growth problems, and developmental delay, although they could not draw definitive conclusions about these possible links. The evidence, however, did suggest that antidepressants raised the rates of miscarriage, low birth weight, transient neonatal symptoms, and persistent pulmonary hypertension of the newborn.

Having weighed the evidence, the researchers concluded the following:

- Adequate treatment of depression is essential, ideally beginning before conception.
- Women with severe recurrent major depression who stop pharmacotherapy are at a high risk for relapse.
- Psychotherapy (preferably cognitive-behavioral therapy or interpersonal psychotherapy) is recommended for treatment of mild to moderate depression during pregnancy.
- Clinicians and patients should make decisions about pharmacotherapy collaboratively.
- Electroconvulsive therapy is an option for severe depression.
- Patients with severe depression, acute suicidality, psychosis, or bipolar disorder should receive psychiatric referrals.

  Clearly, any woman suffering from clinical depression who has been taking SSRIs to manage her condition needs to consult with her physician about weighing the risks and benefits of continuing or discontinuing her medication. For milder, often situational or stress-related depression, however, lifestyle choices can help. These include consuming more omega-3 fatty acids, engaging in physical activity, socializing with friends, getting more sleep, or even taking a yoga or tai chi class.

- **Antipsychotic drugs.** These medications may be necessary for women suffering from schizophrenia and other psychotic illnesses, but they have potent effects on the development of various brain chemicals, especially dopamine. They can also produce long-lasting changes in neurochemistry, brain architecture, and behavior.
- **Terbutaline.** Sold under a variety of brand names, terbutaline is used to treat the symptoms of asthma, bronchitis, and

emphysema. However, its use during pregnancy may lead to an increased incidence of autism spectrum disorders in children, and animal studies suggest that such use might increase the toxic consequences for both mother and child of pesticide exposure in the future.

- **Acetaminophen (Tylenol).** A study involving three hundred African American and Dominican children living in New York City found that children who were exposed to acetaminophen prenatally were more likely to exhibit asthma symptoms at age five. However, the researchers also found that the relationship was stronger when the children had a variant in a particular gene that is involved in the body's ability to detoxify foreign substances and that is common in black and Hispanic populations. In a similar study conducted in Britain, the frequency of Tylenol use during pregnancy and the magnitude of correlation was similar to that found in this study.

Why You Shouldn't Smoke Cigarettes or Drink Alcohol

I'm sure you know why you shouldn't smoke cigarettes at all or drink alcohol in excess, but when you're pregnant, your smoking and drinking are harming your baby as well as yourself. You may have heard that you should not smoke or drink during pregnancy, but you may not be sure exactly why or what problems smoking and drinking can cause.

Smoking

The substances you inhale when you're smoking cigarettes—including nicotine, lead, arsenic, and carbon monoxide—pass through the placenta and prevent the fetus from getting the proper supply of oxygen and nutrients it needs to grow. According to the

American Lung Association, smoking during pregnancy is estimated to be responsible for 20 to 30 percent of low–birth weight babies, 14 percent of preterm deliveries, and 10 percent of infant deaths.

Premature birth and/or low birth weight puts your baby at risk for long-term disabilities, including cerebral palsy, mental retardation, and learning problems. You also have an increased risk of ectopic pregnancy, vaginal bleeding, placental abruption, and placenta previa (when the placenta covers the opening to the birth canal).

In addition, babies born to women who smoke during pregnancy have a higher rate of cleft lip or palate. And research has shown that male babies in particular may have problems with coordination and physical control because of the way cigarette smoke interacts with testosterone. And if that weren't enough for boys to deal with, research also indicates that smoking (along with alcohol consumption) during pregnancy may be harmful to the developing testicles and increase the risk for male reproductive problems.

Even if you don't smoke, your exposure to secondhand smoke may also affect your baby. At least one study has found evidence linking pregnant women's secondhand smoke exposure to their children's ADHD, aggressiveness, defiance, and conduct disorder, including truancy, fighting, school failure, rule breaking, substance abuse, stealing, and property destruction.

So if your partner is a smoker, now is the time to get him to quit!

And other research (see chapter 2) has shown that the inhalation of *any* kind of smoke—be it marijuana, herbal cigarettes, vehicle exhaust, or even the smoke from a barbecue grill—is damaging to the lungs and therefore potentially harmful to your baby.

Drinking

You may have heard that having one or two alcoholic drinks a day can help to reduce your risk for heart attack, and that having a glass of red wine can help to improve your health and increase your longevity. However, people who exercise, eat adequate amounts of fruits and vegetables, do not smoke, and successfully control their weight do not receive any additional health benefit from alcohol. But during pregnancy, it does have significant detrimental effects on the developing fetus from the moment of conception.

The legal drinking age may be twenty-one in most of the United States, but if you drink when you're pregnant, you're giving alcohol to a minor, because your baby is drinking right along with you. And while your body is able to manage the alcohol in your blood, your baby's little liver can't handle it, which is why the alcohol you drink when you're pregnant is much more harmful to your fetus than it is to you.

In addition to causing low birth weight and preterm delivery, your drinking can cause your baby to be born with defects of the heart, brain, and other organs as well as vision or hearing problems, learning disabilities, speech and language delays, and behavioral problems. In fact, studies published to date provide evidence that there is a programming effect on the brain's natural reward circuitry that, at least in some instances, leads to early drinking in the offspring of women who drink during pregnancy. There is also emerging evidence that in high doses, the mother's alcohol consumption raises the risk for the development of all kinds of addictions in her children.

At the most serious end of the potential disability spectrum is fetal alcohol syndrome, which causes permanent damage to the central nervous system, especially to the brain. Developing brain cells and structures can be malformed or have their development interrupted, creating a number of primary cognitive and functional problems. According to an article published in the journal *Lancet*, fetal alcohol syndrome is the leading cause of mental retardation in the Western world. And because brain development is ongoing throughout gestation, alcohol exposure presents a risk of fetal brain damage at any point during pregnancy.

Choose to Be Physically Active

Physical activity, like smoking, drinking, and taking recreational drugs, is a lifestyle choice, so make the healthy choice and get sufficient physical activity throughout your pregnancy. At any time of life, but particularly during pregnancy, regular physical activity will regulate your blood sugar, control your blood pressure, and elevate your mood. It will generally create a healthier physical environment for your developing baby.

Unfortunately, less than 25 percent of pregnant women are now getting the amount of physical activity recommended by the government. ACOG calls for women with uncomplicated pregnancies to get thirty minutes or more of moderate exercise on most days, and the Department of Health and Human Services recommends two and a half hours of moderate aerobic activity each week during pregnancy.

Although the connection between exercise and control of blood sugar (which is particularly important during pregnancy) may not seem immediately obvious, it lies in the fact that muscle is the primary regulator of blood sugar; in addition, excess blood sugar (glucose) is stored in muscle tissue in the form of glycogen. So the less muscle you have, the harder it is for your body to control your blood sugar. Too much glucose in the blood leads to an increased risk of diabetes.

Thus, getting more exercise works to reduce the risk of diabetes two ways: by reducing your blood sugar level and by helping to control your weight. Even starting with ten minutes a day and gradually working up to thirty minutes, five days a week, will help. It has been shown that for most people, simply losing ten to fourteen pounds, or 10 percent of their excess weight, will make a real difference in their blood sugar levels. Of course, when you are pregnant, you should not be losing weight unless you are under the close supervision of a health-care professional. It's preferable to lose the weight before becoming pregnant. This is not to say, however, that you should not be physically active.

In terms of mood, regular physical activity has been shown to reduce stress, ward off anxiety and feelings of depression, boost self-esteem, and improve sleep. The reason is brain chemistry. When you exercise, your body releases chemicals called endorphins, which interact with the receptors in your brain that reduce your perception of pain. Endorphins also trigger a positive feeling in the body similar to that of morphine. For example, the feeling that follows a run or a workout is often described as a "runner's high," which is accompanied by a positive and energizing outlook on life. For that reason, exercise is an effective treatment for mild to moderate depression.

In addition, a few studies have looked at the relationship between changes in physical activity and changes in mood and have found that low physical activity was correlated with higher scores in anxiety and depression.

ACOG considers brisk walking, swimming, cycling, and aerobic classes safe during uncomplicated pregnancies, even for women who have not exercised regularly before becoming pregnant. Running, racquet sports, and strength training are also safe in moderation for women who have regularly engaged in them before pregnancy. Activities that are not recommended include downhill skiing, contact sports, and scuba diving.

ACOG also recommends that women who have not exercised regularly before becoming pregnant start slowly and build up to thirty minutes a day minimum. Of course, everyone should always consult with her doctor before beginning any kind of exercise program. Always wear comfortable clothing and a bra that fits well and gives lots of support, and be sure to drink plenty of water. After the first trimester, you should avoid exercising while lying on your back, in hot humid weather, or when you have a fever. Stop exercising if you experience vaginal bleeding, dizziness, chest pain, headache, muscle weakness, calf pain or swelling, uterine contractions, decreased fetal movement, or fluid leaking from the vagina.

Here are some physical activity websites that can help you to get started and keep you moving:

http://www.walkfithealth.com
http://www.6Levels.com
http://myfitnesspal.com/

Get a Good Night's Sleep

Sleep deprivation is known to increase blood sugar and blood pressure, contribute to weight gain and stress, and elevate inflammation at the cellular level.

Newborns sleep between sixteen and eighteen hours out of every twenty-four hours; by six months of age, babies sleep about fourteen hours out of twenty-four, and adults should optimally be getting between seven and eight and a half hours of sleep every night. There is an inverse relationship between hours of sleep and levels of high-sensitivity C-reactive protein (hs-CRP), an inflammatory marker that can easily be measured. People who averaged four hours of sleep per night for ten days had hs-CRP markers correlated with an increased rate of cardiovascular disease. In general, multiple inflammatory markers go up when sleep decreases to less than seven hours. Even coronary artery calcification is related to a lack of sleep.

A study of twenty-one thousand twins over twenty-two years showed that when adults slept less than an average of seven hours a night, the men's rate of dying in that period increased by 26 percent, and the women's by 21 percent. A 2003 study published in the *Journal of the American Medical Association* showed that women who slept less than seven hours a night had a higher rate of coronary "events" than those who slept eight hours. And the rate increased threefold for those who slept less than five hours at least twice a week.

Many of the adverse results of sleep deprivation are related to disruptions in proper hormone function, a lowering of glucose regulatory mechanisms and insulin secretion even in otherwise healthy people.

In one study, healthy people who experienced twenty-four hours of sleep deprivation had a significant increase in their steady state glucose (SSG) level. People with insulin resistance have a higher SSG, and insulin resistance is an early sign of the development of type 2 diabetes. Many investigators now think that chronic sleep loss may contribute to the development of type 2 diabetes and also be at least partly responsible for the obesity epidemic in the United States and, increasingly, throughout the developed world.

Sleep deprivation may also increase the stress hormone cortisol, and chronically elevated cortisol secretion has been linked to obesity and diabetes. In one study, elevated cortisol levels in women were correlated with increased calorie intake and an increased consumption of sugary foods. In another study, a group of healthy men showed a 37 percent increase in cortisol after sleeping for only four hours, and those who were totally deprived of sleep showed a 45 percent increase. Cortisol stimulates the breakdown of muscle protein, which in turn contributes to elevated blood glucose and may also contribute to lowering metabolism (because muscle burns calories more quickly than fat does). The result is a higher blood sugar level and increased body weight.

LOWER CORTISOL BY DRINKING GREEN TEA

Green tea has been shown to lower the cortisol level, so if you're feeling stressed, make yourself a nice cup of Dr. Steve's Green Tea (see chapter 1).

To top it all off, lack of sleep also influences the hormones that are known to affect appetite and control energy balance (that is, calories in versus calories out). Leptin is a hormone secreted from fat tissue that binds to the receptors in the hypothalamus, which is the appetite-control center of the brain. In general, the leptin level is higher with higher body fat and recent feeding; therefore, a high leptin level signals your brain that you are full. In a study of eleven lean men, sleeping only four hours a night caused a 20 percent drop in the circulating leptin, independent of changes in fat mass or energy intake. Therefore, a lack of sleep signals the body that the energy level is low.

Ghrelin is a hormone secreted by the stomach that tells your body it needs energy (food). A study has shown that only one night of total sleep deprivation induced a 22 percent increase in the circulating ghrelin level and increased hunger in nine healthy men. Another study of twelve healthy men subjected to two four-hour nights of sleep showed that sleep loss was correlated with a decrease in leptin, an increase in circulating ghrelin, and increased hunger. Needless to say, this is a combination destined to lead to overeating.

In a study of normal-weight adults and children, those who got six hours of sleep a night had a 23 percent higher rate of being overweight than those who got seven to eight hours of sleep. Those who slept five hours had a 40 percent higher rate of obesity, and the ones who got four hours or less had a 73 percent rate.

Yet another study looked at thirty normal-weight men and women who slept either nine or four hours a night for six nights in a row. After each sleep session their brains were evaluated with magnetic resonance imaging. The results suggested a correlation between sleep restriction and obesity because of neuronal activity when the participants were exposed to food stimuli. Apparently, restricted sleep affected parts of the brain that are linked to motivation and desire and that may be related to an increased propensity to seek food. This particular study did not distinguish between high- and low-calorie foods, but other studies suggest that high-calorie foods may be preferred by those who experience sleep restriction, and there is compelling evidence that snack-food consumption increases during periods of sleep restriction.

• •

Dr. Steve's Bedtime Snack

Tryptophan, an amino acid found in high concentrations in dairy products as well as turkey, is essential for the production of serotonin, a brain chemical that has sleep-inducing qualities. Milk has even been called "sleep juice." So for a sleep-inducing bedtime snack, have a glass of warm, organic, nonfat milk with a small amount of dark honey and a piece of whole-grain bread. The carbs in the bread will enable your body to use the tryptophan in the milk for manufacturing serotonin instead of for some other purpose.

• •

Aside from affecting weight issues, sleep deprivation and stress seem to create a vicious cycle. If, as we have seen, lack of sleep elevates the stress hormone cortisol, then sleep deprivation contributes to feelings of stress. In addition, the amount of sleep we get (or don't get) is directly related to elevated blood levels of C-reactive protein and other inflammatory markers, independent of any other lifestyle or nutritional choices we might make. So when we're stressed, we don't sleep well, and when we don't sleep well, our stress levels go up—and the cycle continues.

In a nutshell, the formula for having the healthiest baby possible seems to be the following: eat a nutritious SuperFoods diet, keep your environment as toxin-free as possible, get enough physical exercise, and get enough sleep. You'll maintain a healthy weight and avoid a multitude of potential health problems for both you and your baby.

Some Tips for Getting More Sleep

- Try to become a good sleeper before you get pregnant, even if it means seeing a sleep specialist.
- Never argue in bed (or in the bedroom, for that matter.) Try to settle problems early in the day.

- Eat dinner at least three hours before bedtime and go to bed a little bit hungry—or at least not stuffed.
- Eat foods containing melatonin. (See below.)
- Take a warm bath or shower at bedtime. It will relax you, and the rapid drop in body temperature afterward has a sleep-inducing benefit.
- Be sure that your bedroom is comfortable, dark, and quiet.
- Give your bedmate a back rub, a hand rub, a foot rub, or a neck rub; it will relax both of you and you'll sleep better. It takes my wife less than five minutes to put me to sleep using one of these "rubs."
- Get a red nightlight so that you don't have to turn on a white light if you get up to go to the bathroom. White light (as well as any artificial light in the blue-light spectrum, such as computer screens and fluorescent bulbs) stops the production of melatonin, so that when you get back to bed, your brain has to start all over again.
- Get a lavender-scented candle, but be sure it's natural lavender, not an artificial fragrance that may bring toxic phthalates into your bedroom.
- Don't drink caffeinated coffee within three or four hours of going to bed.
- Reduce the sodium in your diet. Sodium isn't good for you, anyway, but a high-salt diet also impairs sleep.

· ·

How Food Induces Sleep

Melatonin is manufactured by the pineal gland and in the gastro-intestinal tract. This potent antioxidant and immune-system booster plays a major role in synchronizing our circadian rhythms and thus helps to induce sleep.

Melatonin is found in walnuts and tart cherries and, to a lesser degree, in grape skins, tomatoes, rice, and oats. Although lower levels of melatonin are found in the blood from consuming melatonin-rich foods than from taking a standard melatonin sleep-aid pill, food sources can help you to establish and maintain a more restful, health-promoting sleep pattern. We need more published scientific papers on this topic, but we already know that cherries, grapes, raisins, oats, rice, and walnuts provide many health benefits for both mother and infant (via breast milk), so consume, enjoy, and hope that it will also benefit your sleep.

• •

7

The Pregnancy Nutrition Program: What, How Much, How Often

This chapter tells you what foods to eat during pregnancy, along with the quantities and the frequency, to maximize the long-term health of both you and your baby. Again, the foods in the tables are listed in order of those that provide the most to those that provide the least. Keep in mind the following:

- Continue eating all of the SuperFoods I recommended in part one.
- Remember that overeating will cause excessive weight gain.
- Be mindful of the number of calories you take in each day.

SuperFood Protein Sources for Pregnant Women

The recommended intake of protein for pregnant or lactating women is about 71 grams per day. Although most people assume that they are eating enough protein, the National Health and Nutrition Survey of 2003–2004 reported that 7.7 percent of adolescent girls and about 8 percent of older females were not meeting the minimum RDA for protein. I recommend that you meet your daily protein requirements by eating a wide range of the following healthy protein sources:

- Jennie-O Ground Turkey Breast Extra Lean (1.5 grams of fat per serving): 26 grams of protein per 3.5 ounces, 120 calories, 70 milligrams of sodium (http://www.switchtoturkey.com)
- Eating Right Boneless Skinless Chicken Breasts: 26 grams of protein per 3.5 ounces, 130 calories, 75 milligrams of sodium (http://www.vons.com/eating right)
- Wild Pacific Salmon Fillet-King (Chinook flash-frozen fillet): 26 grams of protein per 3.5 ounces, 179 calories, 47 milligrams of sodium (http://www.vitalchoice.com)
- Wild Pacific Blue Mussels (flash-frozen): 24 grams of protein per 3.5 ounces, 172 calories, 369 milligrams of sodium (http://www.vitalchoice.com)
- Wild and Pure Alaskan Sockeye Salmon (with skin and bones, BPA-free canned): 23 grams of protein per 3.75 ounces, 160 calories, 359 milligrams of sodium (or 161 calories and 75 milligrams of sodium in the "no salt added" variety) (http://www.vitalchoice.com)
- Wild Pacific Silver Coho Salmon Fillet (flash-frozen): 22 grams of protein per 3.5 ounces, 146 calories, 46 milligrams of sodium (http://www.vitalchoice.com)

- Wild Pacific Red Sockeye Salmon Fillet (flash-frozen): 21 grams of protein per 3.5 ounces, 168 calories, 47 milligrams of sodium (http://www.vitalchoice.com)
- Alaskan Halibut Fillet (flash-frozen): 21 grams of protein per 3.5 ounces, 110 calories, 54 milligrams of sodium (http://www.vitalchoice.com)
- Solgar Whey to Go Whey Protein Powder Natural Vanilla (rBST-free): 20 grams of protein per scoop, 90 calories, 40 milligrams of sodium (http://www.solgar.com)
- Wild and Pure Alaskan Sockeye Salmon (skinless and boneless, BPA-free canned): 19 grams of protein per 3.75 ounces, 133 calories, 359 milligrams of sodium (or 134 calories and 67 milligrams of sodium in the "no salt added" variety) (http://www.vitalchoice.com)
- Voskos Greek Nonfat Yogurt: 15 grams of protein per 5.3-ounce container, 90 calories, 55 milligrams of sodium (http://www.voskos.com)
- King Oscar Sardines in extra-virgin olive oil: 14 grams of protein per 3.75 ounces, 240 calories, 300 milligrams of sodium (http://www.kingoscar.com)
- Kirkland Wild Alaskan Sockeye Salmon (BPA-free canned): 12 grams of protein per ¼ cup, 60 calories, 230 milligrams of sodium (http://www.costco.com)
- Julian Bakery Low Carb Smart Carb #1 (a complete sprouted high-protein bread): 12 grams of protein per slice, 9 calories, 140 milligrams of sodium (http://www.julianbakery.com)
- Horizon Organic Fat-Free Milk: 9 grams of protein per cup, 90 calories, 120 milligrams of sodium (http://www.horizonorganic.com)
- Häagen-Dazs Vanilla All Natural Low-Fat Frozen Yogurt: 9 grams of protein per ½ cup, 180 calories, 45 milligrams of sodium (http://www.haagendazs.com)

- Horizon Organic DHA Omega-3 Fat-Free Milk: 9 grams of protein per cup, 100 calories, 160 milligrams of sodium (http://www.horizonorganic.com)

- Cascade Fresh Nonfat Yogurt: 10 grams of protein per 6 ounces, 80 calories, 110 milligrams of sodium (http://www.cascadefresh.com).

- Lactaid Lactose-Free Nonfat Yogurt: 7 grams of protein per cup, 140 calories, 120 milligrams of sodium (1-800-522-TAID)

- Stonyfield Organic 0% Fat Yogurt: 7 grams of protein per cup, 100 calories, 120 milligrams of sodium (http://www.stonyfield.com).

- Yoplait Original 99% Fat-Free Low-Fat Yogurt: 5 grams of protein per container, 170 calories, 85 milligrams of sodium (http://www.yoplait.com)

- Westbrae Natural Vegetarian Organic Lentil Beans: 8 grams of protein per ½ cup, 100 calories, 150 milligrams of sodium (1-800-434-4246)

- MaraNatha Organic Roasted Peanut Butter: 8 grams of protein per 2 tablespoons, 180 calories, 0 milligrams of sodium (http://www.maranathafoods.com)

- MaraNatha Natural Almond Butter: 7 grams of protein per 2 tablespoons, 190 calories, 0 milligrams of sodium (http://www.maranathafoods.com)

- Kirkland Organic Vanilla Soymilk: 6 grams of protein per cup, 100 calories, 95 milligrams of sodium (http://www.costco.com)

- 365 Organic Soymilk: 6 grams of protein per cup, 90 calories, 110 milligrams of sodium (http://www.wholefoodsmarket.com)

- Silk All Natural Soymilk: 7 grams of protein per cup, 100 calories, 120 milligrams of sodium (http://www.silk.com)

Foods That Control Blood Sugar

Beans (all)	4 ½-cup servings per week
Whole grains (all)	3 to 4 servings or 10 grams per day
Apples (and pears, bananas, and pineapple)	1 medium per day
Honey (preferably dark)	1 to 2 tablespoons daily
Peanut butter (natural, unsalted)	2 tablespoons 5 times per week

For some of my favorite peanut butter choices, see chapter 11.

Nuts (raw or dry-roasted, unsalted)	1 oz 5 times per week
Almonds (raw)	24 nuts
Almonds (dry-roasted)	22 nuts
Walnuts	7 nuts
Hazelnuts (raw)	20 nuts
Peanuts (dry-roasted, unsalted)	48 nuts
Pecans (raw)	10 nuts
Pistachios (dry-roasted, unsalted)	47 kernels
Jumbo cashews (dry-roasted)	15 nuts

One salted cashew that passes my inspection even though it is salted is Planters Jumbo Cashews, dry-roasted in sea salt. They have only 100 milligrams of sodium per serving of fifteen nuts (http://www.planters.com, 1-877-677-3268).

Sources of Vitamin A

The Recommended Daily Allowance (RDA) for vitamin A for males fourteen years and older is 900 micrograms per day; for females fourteen years and older, it's 700 micrograms daily.

The RDA for pregnant women eighteen years and younger is 750 micrograms; for pregnant women nineteen years and older, it is 770 micrograms daily. For breast-feeding women, the RDA is

1,200 micrograms for those eighteen and under, and 1,300 micrograms for those nineteen and older.

Preformed Vitamin A

Egg (1 large)	84–119 mcg
Milk, fortified (8 oz)	76–150 mcg
Cheddar cheese (1 oz)	90 mcg

Carotenoid (Plant) Sources of Vitamin A

Beta-Carotene

Aim for 6 milligrams daily from a combination of the following.

Sweet potato (1 cup cooked)	23 mg
Carrot juice (1 cup)	22 mg
Pumpkin, canned (1 cup)	17 mg
Carrots (1 cup cooked and sliced)	13 mg
Spinach (1 cup cooked)	11.3 mg
Kale (1 cup cooked and chopped)	10.6 mg
Butternut squash (1 cup cooked and cubed	9.4 mg
Collard greens (1 cup cooked and chopped)	9.2 mg
Pumpkin pie (1 slice)	7.4 mg
Cantaloupe (1 cup cubed)	3.2 mg
Apricot, fresh (3)	1.6 mg
Apricot, dried (¼ cup)	1.4 mg

Alpha-Carotene

Aim for a total of 2.4 millgrams daily from a combination of the following.

Pumpkin, canned (1 cup)	11.7 mg
Carrots (1 cup cooked and sliced)	6.6 mg
Baby carrots, raw (10)	3.8 mg
Orange bell pepper (1 large)	0.3 mg
Collard greens (1 cup cooked and chopped)	0.2 mg

Beta-Cryptoxanthin

Aim for 1 milligram daily from a combination of the following.

Butternut squash (1 cup cooked and cubed)	9.4 mg
Red bell pepper strips (1 cup cooked)	2.8 mg
Japanese persimmon (1)	2.4 mg
Papaya (1 cup mashed)	1.8 mg
Red bell pepper, raw (1 large)	0.8 mg
Tangerine juice (1 cup)	0.5 mg
Tangerine (1 medium)	0.3 mg

Sources of Vitamin K

The Adequate Intake (AI) for vitamin K for males fourteen to eighteen is 75 micrograms daily; for men nineteen and older, the value is 120 micrograms daily.

The AI recommended by the Institute of Medicine for vitamin K from all sources is 75 micrograms per day for pregnant and breast-feeding women eighteen and younger and 90 micrograms for those nineteen and older.

Kale (1 cup chopped and raw)	547 mcg
Swiss chard (1 cup chopped and raw)	299 mcg
Parsley (¼ cup raw)	246 mcg
Spinach (1 cup raw)	145 mcg
Leaf lettuce (1 cup shredded)	118 mcg
Soybean oil (1 tbsp)	25 mcg
Canola oil (1 tbsp)	20 mcg
Broccoli (1 cup cooked and chopped)	20 mcg

Sources of Calcium

The Recommended Daily Allowance (RDA) for calcium for males and females fourteen to eighteen is 1,300 milligrams per day. For adult men and women nineteen to fifty, it's 1,000 milligrams, and for those fifty-one and older, the value is 1,200 milligrams daily.

For pregnant and breast-feeding women ages eighteen years and under, the RDA is 1,300 milligrams per day; for those nineteen and older, it is 1,000 milligrams.

Food	Quantity of Calcium	Percentage of Calcium Absorbed
Sesame seeds (¼ cup)	351 mg	unknown
Cheddar cheese (1.5 oz)	303 mg	32%
Milk (8 oz)	300 mg	32%
Yogurt (8 oz)	300 mg	32%
Tofu (½ cup cubed)	258 mg	31%
Rhubarb (½ cup chopped)	174 mg	9%
Spinach (½ cup cooked)	115 mg	5%
White beans (½ cup cooked)	115 mg	22%
Collard greens (½ cup cooked and chopped)	113 mg	unknown
Bok choy (½ cup cooked and chopped)	79 mg	54%
Kale (½ cup cooked and chopped)	61 mg	49%
Orange (1)	52 mg	unknown
Broccoli (½ cup cooked and chopped)	35 mg	61%

Adapted from: J. Higdon, *An Evidence-Based Approach to Vitamins and Minerals* (Stuttgart, Germany: Thieme, 2003).

Sources of Iron

The Recommended Daily Allowance (RDA) for iron for males fourteen to eighteen is 11 milligrams per day; for men nineteen and older, it's 8 milligrams daily. The RDA for females fourteen to eighteen is 15 milligrams per day; for women nineteen and older, it's 8 milligrams daily. For pregnant women of all ages, the value is 27 milligrams per day. For breast-feeding women eighteen and younger, the RDA is 10 milligrams per day; for women nineteen and older, it's 9 milligrams daily.

Tofu (4 oz)	6.1 mg
Bran cereal with raisins (1 cup)	5 mg
Oysters (6 medium)	5 mg
Soybeans (½ cup)	4.4 mg
Lean beef tenderloin, grass-fed (4 oz)	4 mg
Quinoa (¼ cup)	3.9 mg
Blackstrap molasses (1 tbsp)	3.5 mg
Lentils (½ cup cooked)	3.3 mg
Spinach (½ cup cooked)	3.2 mg
Prune juice (¾ cup)	2.3 mg
Kidney beans (½ cup cooked)	2.6 mg
Cashews (1 oz)	1.7 mg
Turkey breast (3 oz)	1.6 mg
Shrimp, cooked (8 large)	1.4 mg
Chicken, dark meat (3 oz)	1.1 mg
Prunes (5, or 1.5 oz)	1 mg
Raisins (1 small box)	0.89 mg

Sources of Magnesium

The Recommended Daily Allowance (RDA) for magnesium for males fourteen to eighteen is 410 milligrams per day; for men nineteen to thirty, it's 400 milligrams, and for those thirty-one and older, it's 420 milligrams daily.

The RDA for females fourteen to eighteen is 360 milligrams per day; for women nineteen to thirty, it's 310 milligrams, and for those thirty-one and older, it's 320 milligrams daily.

The RDA for pregnant women eighteen and younger is 400 milligrams; for pregnant women nineteen to thirty, it's 350 milligrams; and for those thirty-one and older, it's 360 milligrams. For breast-feeding women eighteen and younger, the RDA is 360 milligrams; for breast-feeding women nineteen to thirty, it's 310 milligrams; and for those thirty-one and older, it's 320 milligrams.

Pumpkin seeds (¼ cup)	185 mg
Spinach (1 cup cooked)	156 mg
Swiss chard (1 cup chopped and cooked)	150 mg
Soybeans (1 cup cooked)	147 mg
Green beans (1 cup cooked)	140 mg
Wild Chinook salmon (4 oz)	138 mg
100% bran (e.g., All Bran) cereal (½ cup)	128 mg
Sunflower seeds (¼ cup)	127 mg
Black beans (1 cup cooked)	120 mg
Oat bran, dry (½ cup)	96 mg
Pinto beans (1 cup cooked)	94 mg
Cashews (¼ cup)	89 mg
Brown rice (1 cup cooked)	83 mg
Almonds, raw or dry-roasted (22, or 1 oz)	81 mg
Ground flaxseed meal (2 tbsps)	70 mg
Lima beans (½ cup cooked)	63 mg
Shredded wheat (2 pieces)	54 mg
Peanuts (1 oz)	50 mg
Hazelnuts (1 oz)	49 mg
Quinoa (½ cup cooked)	45 mg
Buckwheat (½ cup cooked)	44 mg
Black-eyed peas (½ cup cooked)	43 mg
Blackstrap molasses (1 tbsp)	43 mg
Yellow squash (1 cup cooked)	43 mg
Broccoli (1 cup cooked)	39 mg
Banana (1 medium)	34 mg
Milk (8 oz)	34 mg
Tofu (4 oz)	34 mg

Sources of Chromium

The Adequate Intake (AI) of chromium for males fourteen to fifty is 35 micrograms per day; for men fifty-one and older, it's 30 micrograms daily.

The Recommended Daily Allowance (RDA) for females fourteen to eighteen is 24 micrograms per day; for women nineteen to fifty, it's 25 micrograms, and for women fifty-one and older, it's 20 micrograms daily. The AI of chromium for pregnant women eighteen and younger is 29 micrograms per day; for pregnant women nineteen and older, it's 30 micrograms. For breast-feeding women eighteen and younger, it's 44 micrograms, and for breast-feeding women nineteen and older, it's 45 micrograms.

The problem with getting chromium from food sources, however, is that the amount varies from batch to batch and depends where the food was grown, so the best way to be sure you're getting the right amount is to take it in supplement form (see chapter 12).

Onion (1 cup)	25 mcg
Romaine lettuce (2 cups, shredded)	16 mcg
Broccoli (½ cup chopped and cooked)	11 mcg
Tomato (1 cup chopped)	9 mcg
Grape juice (8 oz)	7.5 mcg

Dr. Steve's Thirteen Easy Ways to Give Your Body a Potassium Boost

The 2010 Dietary Guidelines for Americans (http://www.cnpp.usda.gov/publications/dietaryguidelines/2010policydoc/policydoc.pdf) lists the AI for potassium at 4,700 milligrams per day. It does not break down the values by age or sex. But I suggest that, like our Paleolithic ancestors, you aim for about 8,000 milligrams per day from food.

Swiss chard (1 cup chopped and cooked)	960 mg
Sweet potato (1 cup cooked)	950 mg
Spinach (1 cup cooked)	838 mg
Papaya (1 medium)	781 mg
Carrot juice (1 cup)	640 mg
Sunsweet Prune Juice (1 cup)	540 mg
R. W. Knudsen Very Veggie Vegetable juice, unsalted (1 cup)	520 mg

Libby's Canned Pumpkin (1 cup)	505 mg
Cantaloupe (1 cup cubed)	494 mg
Naked Juice Just O-J (1 cup)	470 mg
Banana (1 medium)	457 mg
Oats (½ cup cooked)	335 mg
Deglet Noor Dates (6)	324 mg

Sources of Alpha-Linolenic Acid

The Food and Nutrition Board of the National Institute of Medicine has set an Adequate Intake (AI) of 1.6 grams per day of plant-derived omega-3s (alpha-linolenic acid, ALA) for males fourteen and older and 1.1 grams per day for females fourteen and older. The AI for pregnant women of all ages is 1.4 grams per day; for lactating women of all ages, it's 1.3 grams.

Oils

Walnut oil (1 tbsp)	1.4 g
Canola oil (1 tbsp)	1.3 g
Soybean oil (1 tbsp)	0.7 g

Other Foods

Walnuts (7, or 1 oz)	2.6 g
Flaxseed (1 tbsp)	2.2 g
Soy nuts, dry-roasted (½ cup)	1.2 g
Wheat germ (½ cup)	0.5 g
Collard greens (1 cup chopped and cooked)	0.2 g
Spinach (1 cup cooked)	0.2 g
Egg (1 large)	0.15 to 0.25 g

Sources of Choline

The Adequate Intake (AI) of choline is 550 milligrams per day for males fourteen and older and 400 milligrams for females fourteen to eighteen. For women nineteen and older, the AI is 425 milligrams per day.

The AI for all pregnant women is 450 milligrams; for breast-feeding women, it's 550 milligrams.

Data from the 2003–2004 National Health and Nutrition Examination Survey conducted by the CDC found that no more than 10 percent of older children, men, women, and pregnant women had choline intakes at the recommended level. Here is a list of good food sources from the USDA. I also recommend that everyone take a daily choline supplement (see chapter 12).

Egg (1 large)	110 mg
Cod (4 oz)	95 mg
Shrimp (4 oz)	92 mg
Navy beans (1 cup cooked)	82 mg
Salmon (4 oz)	74 mg
Brussels sprouts (1 cup cooked)	64 mg
Broccoli (1 cup chopped and cooked)	63 mg
Pinto beans (1 cup cooked)	62 mg
Kidney beans (1 cup cooked)	60 mg
Cauliflower (1 cup chopped and cooked)	49 mg
Asparagus (1 cup chopped and cooked)	47 mg
Spinach (1 cup cooked)	45 mg
Green peas (1 cup cooked)	44 mg
Corn (1 cup)	36 mg
Buckwheat (1 cup cooked)	34 mg
Tofu (4 oz)	32 mg
Cabbage (1 cup chopped and cooked)	30 mg
Winter squash (any kind, 1 cup cubed and cooked)	22 mg
Cashews (¼ cup)	21 mg
Avocado (1 cup cubed)	21 mg
Peanuts (¼ cup)	19 mg
Almonds (¼ cup)	19 mg

My Twelve Favorite Sources of Betaine

The quantities below are all per 3.5 ounces of food.

Wheat bran	1,507 mg
Wheat germ, toasted	1,396 mg
Spinach, frozen, whole leaf, cooked	809 mg
Uncle Sam Cereal	248 mg
Graham crackers	194 mg
Whole-wheat bread	180 mg
Post Shredded Wheat	158 mg
Barley malt flour	66 mg
Oat bran	36 mg
Sweet potato	35 mg
Shrimp, canned	33 mg
Curry powder	28.8 mg

Sources of Riboflavin

The RDA for riboflavin for males fourteen and older is 1.3 mg per day; for females fourteen to eighteen, it's 1.0 milligrams, and for women nineteen and older, it's 1.1 milligrams.

The RDA for pregnant women of all ages is 1.4 milligrams, and for breast-feeding women, it's 1.6 milligrams.

Nonfat yogurt (1 cup)	0.5 mg
Spinach (1 cup cooked)	0.4 mg
Milk (1 cup)	0.34 mg
Egg (1 large)	0.27 mg
Almonds (1 oz)	0.24 mg
Broccoli (1 cup chopped and cooked)	0.18 mg
Asparagus (6 spears)	0.13 mg
Salmon (3 oz)	0.13 mg
Chicken breast (3 oz)	0.1 mg
Raspberries (1 cup)	0.1 mg

Plum (1)	0.1 mg
Halibut (3 oz)	0.08 mg

Fish Sources of EPA and DHA

For food sources of omega-3, see the chart in chapter 4. I recommend three to four ounces of any of the fish listed there two to four times a week, with one exception: to be perfectly safe, pregnant women should not eat *any* tuna, and men should consume no more than six ounces of tuna a week.

PART 3

The "Fourth Trimester"

You're going to be reading a lot about breast-feeding in this section, especially in chapter 8, because not only I but also many scientists and government agencies, including the World Health Organization, are convinced that this is perhaps the most important thing you can do to ensure your new baby's healthy development and reduce his or her risk for many diseases later in life.

One reason to be as healthy as possible before you give birth is that your newborn will continue to be largely dependent on your immune system while his or hers is still developing. The more normal your weight, blood sugar, and inflammatory markers are during pregnancy, the better the chances that your breast milk will contain the optimum hormone levels for your baby's health at birth and throughout life. Not only will particular compounds in your breast milk (which are not found in formula) help your baby to avoid infections, allergies, and asthmalike symptoms, they will also reduce his or her chances of developing serious autoimmune diseases, including type 1 diabetes. In fact, as you will see, breast-feeding has been shown to protect babies from a wide range of potential diseases and developmental issues, including obesity.

To make sure that you pass along optimum immunity to your child, it is, of course, important that you consume as many health-promoting nutrients as possible through diet and/or supplements, so we'll discuss just which vitamins, minerals, and antioxidants are most important for the baby's health now and for years to come.

Breast-feeding is also good for you. Not only does it speed up the loss of postpregnancy baby weight, it has also been shown to reduce your risk for developing heart disease and breast cancer.

Having a new baby is both joyful and stressful, and there is evidence to show that when breast-feeding is going well, it helps to reduce maternal stress, which has health benefits for both of you.

As with many things in life, there's a synergistic relationship among the chemical reactions in your body related to stress, weight, and sleep. While breast-feeding increases the production of a particular brain chemical associated with good feelings, stress can block the production of this hormone by releasing another that keeps you in a constant state of fight-or-flight and reduces your ability to get a good night's sleep. Lack of sleep can then create more stress and make it harder to control your body weight. In chapter 9 I'll explain all these interactions and offer you some tips for nonmedical ways to reduce stress and get more sleep. I'll also talk about the many important ways that physical activity fits into the mix and helps you to lose weight, boost your mood, and deal with the normal stresses related to mothering a newborn.

Even if there is a health problem that prevents you from breast-feeding, following the rest of the advice in these chapters will help to ensure the optimal health of your newborn as well as your own. I have included two excellent organic infant formulas in chapter 11; of course, you should seek the advice of your health-care professional.

No matter what your personal situation may be, my goal is to leave you, your spouse or partner, and your baby headed down the road to a long, healthy, and fulfilling life.

8

Breast-Feeding Your Baby

Congratulations! You have a beautiful new baby. All you want now is for your baby to be as happy and healthy as possible for the rest of his or her life and for you to be a happy and healthy mom. Don't stop doing all the good things you've already been doing. The goal is to keep your infant's external environment free of harmful substances and his internal environment full of health-promoting nutrients.

Even though we're talking specifically about the benefits of breast-feeding here, it's important to emphasize that dads (as well as other family and close friends) are still involved. Your spouse or partner is also a partner in child rearing and your most important support system during what can be a stressful time in your life. Although he cannot physically feed your infant (except when milk is expressed), he can certainly feed your well-being and that of your child, both emotionally and in practical ways.

I'm sure you've heard that breast milk is the best food you can give your newborn and that the longer you can continue breast-feeding, the better off your baby will be. But you may not have heard that breast-feeding also has significant health benefits for women, both immediately and in the future. In this chapter we'll talk about what recent studies have told us about breast-feeding and how your own nutrition affects the well-being of your baby. Up until now you've been feeding your baby the substances in your blood that are carried to the fetus through the umbilical cord; now you're feeding him or her the substances contained in your breast milk.

Babies were exclusively breast-fed for thousands of years. It is only as formula has become more readily available and societies have become industrialized and affluent that women have even had the ability to choose whether to breast-feed. In fact, in some developing societies, choosing *not* to breast-feed has become a socioeconomic status symbol. Unfortunately, this is one instance in which modernization is not an improvement. The goal of this chapter is to increase your awareness of the many benefits of breast-feeding so that you will be committed to feeding your baby the "old-fashioned" way.

The Many Benefits of Breast Milk

One of the reasons most often given for choosing to breast-feed is that new mothers pass along their own mature immune responses to their babies and provide protection from disease while the newborns' own immune systems are not yet fully developed.

The first month of life is particularly challenging for a newborn's immune system. Emerging from a (we hope) sterile intrauterine environment, the baby is suddenly thrust into a world full of foreign antigens to which he or she has not yet developed an immunity. This leaves the newborn highly susceptible to infections, and infections are the second most common cause of neonatal mortality, accounting for about one million deaths each year worldwide.

The first month of life is therefore the key to developing a well-functioning immune system that will provide a lifetime of good service. In a study of 291 healthy newborns in the Netherlands, the researchers found that exclusive breast-feeding during this time was associated with changing concentrations of white blood cells that mediate and regulate immune responses. The changes were significant enough that by the end of one month, the immune systems of the breast-fed babies were markedly different from, and more efficient than, those of the babies who were not exclusively breast-fed.

The researchers concluded that there are particular compounds found in breast milk but not in formula that modulate the developing immune system to provide more protection from certain infections, asthma, and allergies. For example, a study of more than five thousand children in the Netherlands showed that shorter duration and nonexclusivity of breast-feeding were associated with higher rates of asthma-related symptoms, including wheezing, shortness of breath, dry cough, and persistent phlegm during the children's first four years of life.

A particularly interesting study has shown that breast-fed babies may be protected from developing type 1 diabetes. Unlike type 2 diabetes, in which the body becomes increasingly more resistant to the effects of insulin produced by the pancreas, type 1 is a type of autoimmune disease in which the immune system mistakenly destroys the insulin-producing cells in the pancreas. The incidence of type 1 diabetes has increased dramatically in developed countries in the past several decades, suggesting that nongenetic factors—including dietary changes, increased use of antibiotics, and changes in exposure to infectious diseases—are responsible.

It's also interesting to note that this increase is occurring at the same time that breast-feeding has been decreasing in these countries. Therefore, it would appear that breast-feeding may protect the body from the self-destructive autoimmune responses that can lead to the development not only of type 1 diabetes but also of intestinal disorders, multiple sclerosis, and rheumatoid arthritis as the children get older.

In chapter 3 we discussed the fact that the intestinal microbiomes of lean people have different flora from the microbiomes of people who are overweight. The primary role of your microbiome is to determine the nature and strength of your immune system, and you pass along your immunities to your baby in utero, in the course of a vaginal delivery, and in your breast milk. That's why it's so important for you to clean up your microbiome by eating a variety of SuperFoods even before you become pregnant.

The various bacteria we have in our intestinal tract play a key role in the absorption of nutrients and the protection of our intestines from pathogens. Breast milk provides a continuous source of bacteria to the infant's intestinal tract, and at least one study has shown that the breast milk of the mom and the stool of her infant share some of the same strains of bacteria.

Human milk includes a number of immunological constituents: at least two types of immunoglobins (secretory immunoglobin A and immunoglobin G); free fatty acids; monoglycerides; proteins such as lactoferrin (an important immune system protein that has antibacterial activity in infants) and lactalbumin; glycans (which play an important role in intestinal immunity); nonabsorbed oligosaccharides (carbohydrates that act as prebiotics in the colon); exosomes (small bubbles in the cells that play a role in immune response and cell-to-cell communication), immunomodulators such as cytokines, nucleic acids, and antioxidants; and immune cells such as macrophages, neutrophils, and lymphocytes. All of these interact with one another and with the newborn's intestinal tract, directly or indirectly, to increase immunity to infection, and they probably also contribute to the maturation and efficiency of the newborn immune system.

In one study the researchers found that the mean number of white blood cells in the mothers' milk increased when the babies had an infection and significantly declined between the active infection and convalescence phase. This decline was more significant in the milk of the mothers of the infants with proven localized infections. The mechanism of this phenomenon is not known at this time, but the researchers concluded that their findings support the dynamic immunological connection between lactating mothers and their nursing infants, especially during active infections—thus further encouraging breast-feeding.

Another study showed the thymus glands of breast-fed infants to be twice as large as those of infants who were formula-fed. Since the thymus gland is responsible for producing T-cells (a type of white blood cell), which are an important component of the immune system, this might be one of the ways in which breast-feeding increases immunity.

The transfer of the mother's immune system to her baby begins even before breast-feeding, in the course of vaginal delivery, when the infant is exposed to the mother's vaginal and intestinal flora. Babies born via cesarean section, in contrast, do not have this immune advantage. In addition, it has been shown that women who have C-sections are less likely to breast-feed, thereby further reducing the infant's immunity. C-sections are now the most common surgical procedure done in the United States, accounting for 31.8 percent of all births. There will always be situations in which a C-section is necessary, but elective C-sections are increasing dramatically worldwide. So many factors, socioeconomic and otherwise, seem to be tipping the balance against breast-feeding just when more and more evidence of its many health benefits is emerging.

Breast-feeding also protects babies from gastrointestinal, respiratory, and ear infections. One study suggests that because breast-fed babies are held at a more horizontal angle than those who are bottle-fed, the milk is less likely to run down the auditory canal and into the middle ear; this significantly reduces the chances of a baby's developing infections of the middle ear.

A study done in Britain has shown that babies who were breast-fed for more than four months had greater lung capacity at ten years and eighteen years of age than those who were bottle-fed. The researchers postulated that the greater lung capacity may result from breast-fed babies sucking longer and harder than those who are bottle-fed.

Breast-feeding has also been shown to reduce the rates of serious gastrointestinal diseases (including ulcerative colitis, Crohn's disease, inflammatory bowel syndrome, and celiac disease) and to provide protection from diabetes, lymphoma, leukemia, and Hodgkin's disease when children reach adulthood. Breast-fed babies are less likely to become obese or to have high cholesterol, and they have better cognitive development than babies who are bottle-fed.

One study has shown that children who were breast-fed exclusively for up to three months had IQs that were an average of 2.1 points higher than the IQs of children who were not; children who were breast-fed for four to six months had IQs 2.6 points higher, and those who were breast-fed for more than six months scored 3.8 points higher. This discrepancy was observed by one year of age and held constant throughout the preschool years, when a seven-year follow-up was conducted.

Because our ability to fight disease (that is, the strength of our immune system) depends in large part on our nutritional status, it's important for breast-feeding moms to make sure they are optimizing their own immunity by getting all of the macronutrients, vitamins, minerals, and antioxidants they can through diet. Maternal deficiencies in a variety of nutrients have been shown to have a negative effect on the health of babies who were breast-fed.

• •

Breast-Feeding Improves Outcomes for Preemies

Several studies have shown that premature infants who are breast-fed do better developmentally than those who are formula-fed. One such study, done in Israel and involving four hundred preterm babies (born at thirty-two weeks or less), found that those who were breast-fed had lower rates of necrotizing enterocolitis (a serious condition involving the death of intestinal tissue) and retinopathy of prematurity (a potentially blinding disease in which the retina does not develop normally). Therefore, women whose babies are born prematurely should make every effort to breast-feed their infants to ensure their healthy development.

• •

Vitamins A and D

Adequate levels of vitamins A and D boost intestinal integrity and mucus immune function. The mucous membranes that line the body's cavities and canals (including the intestinal tract, throat, nose, mouth, urethra, rectum, and vagina), produce the mucus that protects them from infection. Your own deficiencies in these micronutrients can cause impaired immune response in your newborn. For SuperFood sources that will boost your levels of vitamins A and D, see chapters 7 and 4, respectively.

• •

Feed Your Baby Carotenoids

Carotenoids are nonvitamin, nonmineral substances that add color to food (such as the orange color of carrots) and have many health benefits, including protection from inflammation, cancer, cardiovascular disease, and eye diseases. Three types of carotenoids—alpha-carotene, beta-carotene, and beta-cryptoxanthin—are the precursors to vitamin A (retinol) and may protect infants from gastrointestinal and respiratory infections.

A study has shown that blood concentrations of carotenoids increase significantly starting two days after birth in breast-fed babies. Therefore, the researchers suggested that the diets of nursing mothers "should include a variety of fruits and veggies to supply a wide spectrum of bioavailable carotenoids to mom and infant."

Another study showed that blood and breast-milk levels of vitamin A increased more after the consumption of fruit than of dark green leafy vegetables and carrots. So the wider the variety of carotenoid-rich SuperFoods you eat, the more health-promoting vitamin A you'll be providing your baby (and yourself).

• •

Vitamin C

Vitamin C is a powerful antioxidant, and Vitamin C deficiency is relatively common, especially among pregnant and breast-feeding women. Because vitamin C is essential for brain development, it's important to make sure your vitamin C status is at an optimum level. Insufficient vitamin C in a newborn can lead to neurological disabilities later in life. Researchers at the University of Copenhagen found that vitamin C deficiency in early postnatal life resulted in impaired neuron development and a functional decrease in spatial memory in guinea pigs, and they speculate that these findings may have clinical implications for children born to vitamin C–deficient mothers.

In addition, it has been shown that the mother's intake of vitamin C from food (much more than from supplements) determined the concentration in her breast milk, and higher concentrations were associated with a 70 percent reduction in the baby's rate of developing allergic reactions. Foods containing vitamin C, including fruits and vegetables, also contain polyphenols, which have been shown by research to work synergistically with vitamin C while also playing a major role in preventing cardiovascular disease and cancer. Furthermore, they are important for gene regulation and expression. So getting your vitamin C from food will benefit both you and your baby.

For a list of foods that are high in vitamin C, see chapter 4.

Vitamin E

Vitamin E affects the body's immune response to allergies. Preliminary studies have shown that it can calm the portions of the immune system that are involved in allergic reactions. Your own higher level of vitamin E will also reduce your baby's allergic sensitivity.

Colostrum, the initial breast milk, has been found to contain about three times more tocopherol than the "mature" (subsequent) milk. Tocopherols are chemical compounds of vitamin E. Thus, there is a large supply of vitamin E during the first week of life, when the infant's own tissue stores are low and need supplementation.

For SuperFood sources of vitamin E, see chapter 4.

Zinc

Zinc deficiency is common during pregnancy, and a nursing mother's zinc deficiency can negatively affect her baby's immune system, leading to acute dermatitis, diarrhea, hair loss, and infections. For SuperFood sources of zinc, see chapter 4. Perinatal maternal zinc supplementation has been shown to improve immune function and neurobehavioral development in the infant.

Iron

Iron is necessary for red blood cells to be able to carry oxygen throughout the body, and iron-deficiency anemia early in life may negatively affect neurochemistry and neurobiology, leading to developmental delays in cognitive and motor functions. To be sure your breast-fed baby is getting enough iron, check out the SuperFood sources in chapter 7. And to ensure that you're receiving the maximum benefit of this important nutrient, eat iron-rich foods in conjunction with foods that are high in vitamin C (for example, four ounces of orange juice with pulp), which will increase the absorption of iron.

In addition to the essential micronutrients discussed above, mother's milk also contains a multitude of bioactive ingredients not found in cow's milk, soy milk, or any other basis of infant formula.

Oligosaccharides

Oligosaccharides are a type of carbohydrate found in many plant foods that work as prebiotics in the colon. They constitute the third largest solid component in human milk, exceeded only by lactose (milk sugar) and lipids. The mother passes oligosaccharides along to her baby in her breast milk, and they then promote the growth and colonization of healthy, good bacteria in the infant's digestive system. Oligosaccharides are found in the urine of breast-fed, but not formula-fed, babies. (For more on prebiotics, see chapter 5.)

In addition to their prebiotic effect, oligosaccharides block the ability of many microorganisms to adhere to the surface of the infant's gastrointestinal tract, thereby protecting him or her from infections and diarrhea. Selectins, a family of molecules involved in cell-to-cell interactions of the immune system, bind to specific oligosaccharides and help white blood cells to reach parts of the body where they might not otherwise be readily available, so that they can do their job of fighting infection and reducing inflammation. Finally, recent discoveries now link oligosaccharides to the promotion of infant brain development.

Plant foods that contain large amounts of oligosaccharides include chicory root, Jerusalem artichokes, onions (including chives, scallions, shallots, and leeks), garlic, legumes, wheat, asparagus, and jicama. So if you increase your intake of these healthy foods, you'll also be boosting your baby's immune system.

Some infant formulas now contain oligosaccharide-like substances. So women who are not breast-feeding—or not exclusively breast-feeding—should discuss the type of formula to use with their doctor.

Beta-Glucans

Beta-glucans are polysaccharides (long carbohydrate molecules) that are known as biological response moderators because of their ability to activate the immune system. They occur most commonly as cellulose in plants, the bran of cereal grains like barley and oats, the cell walls of baker's yeast, certain fungi like shiitake mushrooms, olives, avocados, and bacteria. At least one study has shown a correlation between high beta-glucan exposure and a decreased risk of recurrent wheezing among infants born to parents genetically disposed to be allergic to mold and fungus. So moms need to eat their oatmeal, whole grains, and mushrooms.

• •

Breast-Feeding and Vaccines

Infants who are exclusively breast-fed are less likely to run fevers after their routine immunizations than those who are partly breast-fed or who receive only formula. This may be because breast milk contains anti-inflammatory substances that can reduce fever risk. In addition, immunizations have been shown to work better in babies who are breast-fed. Discuss the specific timing of your baby's immunizations with your health-care provider.

• •

Breast-Feeding, Weight Gain, and Disease Risk Later in Life

We've talked a lot about the relationship between weight and disease, particularly type 2 diabetes and cardiovascular disease. Now there is evidence to show that breast-feeding can protect children from obesity and therefore from the diseases associated with it.

Study after study has shown a difference between breast-fed and formula-fed infants in this regard. By one year old, those who were formula-fed weighed about one pound more than those who were breast-fed. In a 2007 survey of 2,066 Australian boys and girls ages two to sixteen, 22 percent of the boys and 24 percent of the girls were either overweight or obese. The children who had been breast-fed for six months or longer were 36 percent less likely to be overweight and 49 percent less likely to be obese than those who had never been breast-fed.

The unfortunate fact is that several studies now indicate that women with a high prepregnancy BMI (and, consequently, those who are most likely to have overweight or obese children) do not breast-feed for as long a time as women with a normal prepregnancy BMI. One Brazilian study, for example, has shown that women who were overweight or obese and who gained more than the Institute of Medicine's recommendation were two to three times more likely to introduce non–breast milk food and fluids to their infants within one month of birth.

Although the reasons for this discrepancy are unknown and undoubtedly varied, researchers speculate that obese women may have lower prolactin (a hormone that stimulates milk production) levels shortly after delivery and therefore less production of breast milk. They may find it less comfortable to hold their babies for feeding, it may be difficult for the baby to latch on to the breast, they may be uncomfortable with their own body image, or all of the above. This is yet another reason for women to try to take better control of their weight before becoming pregnant.

Rapid weight gain during infancy has been associated with an increased risk for later obesity, and at least one study has shown that formula-fed infants have greater weight gain during infancy than those who are breast-fed. This study found that protein intake was 55 to 80 percent higher in the formula-fed group than in the breast-fed group, and some observational studies have found a higher protein intake during the first two years of life predictive of becoming overweight.

The World Health Organization recommends that infants should be *exclusively* breast-fed until six months of age, and at least one study has concluded that a later introduction of complementary foods was associated with a lower BMI at forty-two years of age, even though there was no statistical difference in BMI during childhood. My own conclusion from these findings is that breast-feeding for six months can protect a child from developing obesity-related diseases later in life.

Yet national statistics from the CDC indicate that only 13.3 percent of women are still breast-feeding exclusively at six months, and only 22.4 percent are breast-feeding at all by twenty to twenty-three months. These figures are disheartening compared to the statistics for breast-feeding worldwide: 37 percent of infants worldwide are breast-fed exclusively for six months, and 39 percent are breast-fed to some extent at twenty to twenty-three months. Although it is understandable that in our industrialized and relatively affluent economy, where most women work outside the home and formula is readily available, societal norms are skewed against long-term breast-feeding, it is unfortunate that the very affluence that should be making us healthier may well be creating the next generation of less healthy adults.

CONSUMER ALERT

Let's encourage employers to make it easier for moms to pump breast milk at work. Ultimately, this may save the employer money by reducing the time mothers take off to nurse a sick infant or child.

It is always possible to find studies that refute the findings of other studies, but the overwhelming evidence indicates that breast-feeding is protective in infancy and throughout life. Breast-fed children may, for example, gain weight faster than formula-fed children during the first two months of life, but they grow more slowly thereafter, and at least one study has shown that rapid weight gain in infancy has less of an effect on body fat percentage, whereas rapid changes in BMI after six months predict, at age four, a higher overall rate of cardiovascular disease later in life.

Thus, ensuring a healthy increase in BMI during the first years of life is a powerful strategy for achieving short- and possibly long-term health. There is a strong link between elevated BMI during childhood and the development of insulin resistance and/or type 2 diabetes in adulthood. In a study that followed children for twenty-six years after their initial recruitment at age nine or ten, the researchers found that those in the top one-fifth for childhood BMI and systolic blood pressure were those most likely to develop type 2 diabetes in young adulthood. Another study, which followed a large cohort of children for more than twenty years, found that 60 percent of those in the top one-fourth of the BMI range at ages nine through eleven remained in the top one-fourth as young adults and had three times the risk of developing type 2 diabetes in adulthood.

Other studies have also shown that breast milk appears to have a protective effect on the development of metabolic disease (including diabetes and obesity), and the evidence suggests that breast-fed infants have lower blood pressure, lower total cholesterol, and lower prevalence of being overweight and obese than those who are bottle-fed.

One of the components of breast milk is a protein called adiponectin, which is involved in regulating the glucose level and in fatty acid breakdown. It is secreted into the bloodstream from fat tissue and from the placenta during pregnancy, and studies have correlated higher blood levels of adiponectin with a lower percentage of body fat. Adiponectin is also known to help suppress the metabolic disruptions that can lead to type 2 diabetes, obesity, atherosclerosis, and nonalcoholic fatty liver disease. Some studies have shown that the higher the level of adiponectin in the breast milk, the lower the breast-fed baby's weight-for-length scores are during the first six months of life. Higher levels of infant adiponectin have also been correlated with lower weight-to-length scores between twelve and twenty-four months.

In terms of long-term protection, a study has shown that adults who were breast-fed in infancy have smaller carotid intima-media thickness and less atherosclerosis at age sixty-five than those who had been formula-fed.

Finally, we know that both young children and adolescents with a higher fitness level also have a healthier cardiovascular profile throughout life. Fitness can reduce the detrimental effects of being overweight and also reduce the risk of becoming overweight in the first place. It's therefore important to note that one study has shown a correlation between a longer duration of breast-feeding and a higher level of fitness independent of birth weight, maternal BMI, or maternal educational level. The researchers concluded that exclusive breast-feeding for three or more months has beneficial effects on cardiovascular health later in life.

Why Is Breast-Feeding So Protective?

Breast milk contains a variety of bioactive substances—including hormones, growth factors, and cytokines (signaling molecules that establish a biochemical communication between mother and child)—that may actively influence the growth and development of the infant. Until recently, the main difference between human milk and commercial formula was considered to be in the fatty acid content—especially omega-6 arachidonic acid and the omega-3 fatty acids EPA and DHA, all of which play a major role in the prevention of central nervous system and cardiovascular disorders.

More recently, however, other bioactive molecules found in breast milk but not in formula are being identified as playing a synergistic, additive, and unique role in human development and health and are, therefore, believed to contribute to the positive effects of breast-feeding. One of the interesting things about all of these factors is that their concentration in breast milk is constantly changing. In other words, a mother's body seems to know when to concentrate what.

The most important of the recently identified protective molecules are the following:

- **Activin-A.** This protein is widely distributed throughout the brain and plays a role in brain recovery from injury as well as central nervous system and cardiac development, and it has been found to influence how well the heart adapts to stress.
- **Follistatin.** This is another neurotropic chemical that works in tandem with activin-A.
- **S100B.** This is a calcium-binding protein mainly concentrated in the central nervous system where it plays a role in cell-to-cell communication, cell growth, cell structure, energy metabolism, and intracellular signaling. Its concentration in breast milk is two hundred times higher than in other biological fluids, such as blood, urine, and spinal fluid.
- **Heme Oxygenase 1.** This is an enzyme that protects the cells from oxidative injury.

The highest concentrations of both activin-A and follistatin have been found in colostrum (the "first" breast milk).

I believe that we will identify more and more protective bioactive molecules in human milk and that it will therefore become even clearer as time goes on why it is so important to breast-feed for as long as possible. I know that it isn't always easy—for any number of reasons that we'll discuss—but I also believe that the more you know about *why* breast-feeding is so important for your child, the more motivated you'll be to make it work for you. That's why I am making it my mission to get the word out.

Breast-Feeding Is Good for the Mother, Too

Losing the baby weight is a high priority for many, if not most, women, and at least one study has shown that for some, breast-feeding may promote postpartum weight loss by increasing energy expenditure by about 450 calories per day. So that's good news!

But if weight loss isn't a great enough incentive to breast-feed, there are other health benefits to consider as well. The choices you make at this time of your life will have consequences for years to come. For example, a twenty-year prospective study funded by the National Institutes of Health found that breast-feeding protected women from developing metabolic syndrome, a predictor of diabetes and heart disease, later in life.

The study showed that among women who did not have gestational diabetes, the risk was lowered by 39 to 56 percent, and for those who did, it was lowered by 44 to 86 percent. This depended on the duration of lactation, which ranged from zero to more than nine months.

Finally, researchers who looked at 60,075 women participating in the Nurses' Health Study II between 1997 and 2005 found a 59 percent reduction in the incidence of premenopausal breast cancer among women who had breast-fed for any length of time and who also had a first-degree relative with breast cancer (which put them at a high risk of developing the disease). The researchers stated that this reduction rate compared favorably to that of hormonal treatments, such as tamoxifen, for women at high risk.

As you'll see in the following chapter, breast-feeding also has stress-reducing, sleep-inducing benefits for both mother and baby. And any new mother can tell you that the less stress and the more sleep you have, the happier and healthier both of you will be. And, happy mom + happy infant = happy dad as well!

9

Sleep, Stress, and Physical Activity

Even though you love your new baby more than anything in the world, the first months of motherhood can be extremely stressful. Your life has really been changed dramatically, and that in itself is stressful. Your sleep patterns have undoubtedly changed (and not for the better), and that too causes stress. Feeling tired adds to your stress, stress makes it more difficult to sleep, and the pattern continues.

In addition, you may be finding it difficult to lose the weight you gained during pregnancy. For a variety of emotional and biochemical reasons, stress and lack of sleep make weight loss more difficult, and if you're not finding time or don't have the inclination to engage in some regular physical activity, that weight will stick around even longer.

In this chapter we're going to discuss the relationship among sleep, stress, and physical activity and offer both scientific explanations and workable solutions to minimize your stress, max-imize your sleep, and fast-track your weight loss so that you can be a happier, healthier mom, both now and in the future.

The Effects of Stress on Breast-Feeding

Studies have shown that stress can affect the production of breast milk, which then affects the mother's ability and/or desire to breast-feed, and that, in turn, can further affect her production of milk.

The production of breast milk occurs in three stages:

1. During the last twelve weeks of pregnancy, the expectant mother's body produces higher levels of prolactin, a hor-mone that stimulates milk production. At the same time the number of prolactin receptors in her breasts, along with the amounts of estrogen and progesterone, increase, which pre-vents the actual production of milk before the baby is born.

2. At birth, the placenta is expelled, causing the mother's estrogen and progesterone levels to drop, thus allowing the prolactin to stimulate her production of milk. When the baby suckles or when the mother pumps breast milk, more prolactin receptors are created in the breasts.

3. The mother now has a mature milk supply, and milk secre-tion is essentially regulated by stimulation of the breast.

Whereas prolactin is important for initiating and maintaining a supply of breast milk, oxytocin is the hormone most closely involved with milk ejection. Oxytocin has been described as the "love" hor-mone because it is secreted during intensely pleasurable experi-ences, such as breast-feeding. Oxytocin is released in short pulses while the baby suckles and is positively correlated with milk volume.

Stress and fatigue increase the production of the stress hor-mone cortisol, decrease oxytocin, and therefore decrease milk production. Less milk may make breast-feeding more stressful and lead to doing it less frequently, which in turn decreases breast stimulation and further reduces milk production. You can see how this quickly becomes a vicious cycle leading to the abandonment of breast-feeding.

At least one study has found that listening to relaxing music before and during breast-feeding has reduced stress and increased milk production. Try it and see if it helps you. If not, try something else. Just don't give up. Breast-feeding in and of itself has been shown to reduce stress, so it may actually become one of the primary tools in your stress-reduction arsenal.

Sleep Is Essential

In *Macbeth*, Shakespeare called sleep the "balm of hurt minds, great nature's second course, chief nourisher in life's feast." And when you had a big test coming up, didn't your mom and your teachers remind you to get a good night's sleep? When you don't get enough sleep, you drag, you're irritable, and you're probably not thinking as clearly as you could be. If you need a refresher course, go back to chapter 6 and reread the section on how a lack of sleep affects your body chemistry.

Those chemical changes affect us both mentally and physically. At least one study has shown that women who reported getting five or less hours of sleep at six months postpartum were 2.3 times more likely to retain at least eleven pounds of pregnancy weight one year after giving birth. That's a substantial amount of weight.

The problem, however, is not just the weight; evidence suggests that compared to women who gain weight at other times, women who retain weight after pregnancy are more likely to remain overweight and tend to deposit it centrally as abdominal fat, which has been linked to a decrease in HDL (good) cholesterol.

A 2010 study published in *Nutrition Today* showed that women who slept a total of at least seven hours sometime during the day and night (that is, not necessarily all at once) were more likely to return to their prepregnancy weight, whereas those who slept less than five hours in a day and night after giving birth were more than twice as likely to retain an extra thirteen pounds of baby weight after one year. In addition, a fifteen-year follow-up study found that 56.3 percent of the women who returned to within 3.3 pounds of their prepregnancy weight by six months postpartum did not become overweight later in life.

A study of both men and women done at the University of Chicago showed that sleeping for 8.5 hours a night, compared to 5.5 hours, while consuming the same amount of food, led to less hunger and a greater loss of fat (with less loss of muscle tissue), even among those who lost the same total amount of weight. The researchers found that when the participants slept for the shorter amount of time, their ghrelin levels increased, and when they slept longer, their levels decreased. Since ghrelin is the hormone that stimulates appetite and fat storage, higher levels could lead to more hunger, greater food intake, and increased weight.

Yet another study has shown that increased ghrelin levels lowered glucose-stimulated insulin secretion, leading to higher levels of circulating blood sugar and a greater rate of diabetes.

So decreased sleep is associated with increased weight, and increased weight is associated with an increased risk for some significant health problems. You may be wondering how, if you're breast-feeding, you can ever expect to get a good night's sleep. And that is, admittedly, an issue. But you may be surprised to learn that at least one Australian study found an increase in slow-wave sleep (deep sleep) in women who breast-fed, compared to those who bottle-fed. The researchers stated that the most likely explanation for the difference was an increase in prolactin levels in the breast-feeding group and suggested that "enhanced SWS [slow-wave sleep] may be another important factor to support breastfeeding in the postnatal period."

Another study found no differences in objective or subjective measures of sleep or sleepiness among mothers who were breast-feeding, those who were formula-feeding, and those who were using a combination of the two. The researchers suggested that even though the breast-feeding mothers might awaken more often, they might also return to sleep more quickly (because they didn't have to get up and prepare a bottle) and not remember the awakenings, or they might actually sleep during the feedings.

Researchers have found that breast milk contains different levels of various nucleotides (molecules that perform a very important role in regulating babies' sleep) at different times of the day and night. The researchers asked a group of women to express milk at different times within a twenty-four-hour period and found that three nucleotides responsible for relaxing the nervous system and promoting restfulness and sleep increased in the samples taken after 8 p.m., peaked in the middle of the night, and lessened in the early morning.

In addition, melatonin, which is manufactured in the adult brain but not the infant brain, reaches its highest concentrations during the night, peaking at 3 a.m., and becomes undetectable in the daytime. Research has shown that babies who receive nocturnal breast milk are less irritable and tend to sleep longer than those who do not.

The point is that breast-feeding can help your baby (and, therefore, you, the mom) sleep better. And if you express milk, you should be giving that milk to your baby at the same time it was expressed.

A small study conducted at the Douglas Hospital Research Centre at McGill University in Montreal, Canada, found that mothers who were breast-feeding reacted less strongly to stress than those who were bottle-feeding. To determine this, the researchers measured cortisol levels in the women's saliva after they had been exposed to stressful situations.

Their conclusion was that breast-feeding had a relaxing or protective effect on the mothers and that this would allow them to "focus more on their children and have more energy for activities such as attending to their infants and producing milk—this is an obvious gain for the children." It is certainly equally beneficial to the mother, since stress negatively affects the life of virtually everyone and is particularly prevalent among women coping with the care of an infant.

• •

Breast-Feeding Is Soothing—Unless It Isn't

We've already discussed the many benefits breast-feeding has for your baby, and now it seems that there are also benefits for you. But it would be untruthful not to point out that for many women, breast-feeding does not come as naturally or as easily as advocates would have you think. And many women simply assume that if they are having difficulty, they are in some way inadequate. They feel ashamed, don't want to ask for help, and therefore abandon breast-feeding for the bottle and deprive both themselves and their baby of a health-promoting and bonding experience.

A study has shown that more than one-third of women experience problems, including pain and nipple cracks, in the first few postpartum days, so it's important to get support and guidance from your doctor or a lactation specialist as soon as possible in order to avoid creating a vicious cycle of difficulty, stress, increased difficulty, and more stress. Stress leads to increased cortisol levels that can in turn lead to imbalances in the immune system. Animal studies have found that a reduction of white blood cells in the mammary glands is correlated to increased stress, and since white blood cells fight infection, this can lead to the development of mastitis (inflammation and/or infection of the breast tissue) or other breast tissue issues.

There are foods that fight infections, and at least one study has shown that raspberries, cranberries, and cloudberries inhibit the growth of staph, E-coli, and salmonella, and are also a natural way to prevent mastitis. And even though there haven't been any studies done on honey in relation to mastitis, we do know that it too inhibits the growth of bacteria, yeast, and fungi.

If you're having a problem breast-feeding, you are far from alone, and you need to get support as quickly as possible. Ask your ob-gyn, talk to the lactation specialist at your hospital (many pediatric practices have a lactation specialist), or contact an organization such as the La Leche League (http://www .llli.org/) to put you in touch with someone in your area who can help.

If you find that you absolutely cannot breast-feed for whatever reason, discuss the alternatives available to you with your health-care provider. Evaluating the pros and cons of one type of formula over another is beyond the scope of this book, and the decision will also depend on the needs of your particular child.

• •

Stress, Sleep, and Postpartum Depression

Several studies have shown that it may be difficult to tell whether someone is depressed or simply tired—especially when that someone is a new mom. Sleep deprivation and stress feed each other, and at a certain point you may not be able to tell whether you're stressed because you're sleep-deprived, sleep-deprived because you're stressed, or actually depressed.

Researchers have found that it's difficult to determine the cause-and-effect relationship between sleep deprivation and postpartum depression, and at least one author has suggested that the latter is simply on a continuum with the former: the less sleep a woman gets, the more likely she is to experience depression. That hypothesis seems to be supported by the evidence that when the baby sleeps better, the mom's depression is alleviated.

Another study, coming at the problem from the opposite direction, concluded, "Women with postpartum depression experienced poorer sleep quality than women without postpartum depression, and sleep quality worsened with increasing postpartum depression symptom severity." The author suggested, "Clinicians need to address measures to improve sleep quality in depressed mothers to decrease symptom severity, and researchers need to develop interventions to facilitate better sleep quality in women with postpartum depression."

A third study found that "poor sleep was associated with depression, independently of other risk factors," and concluded that "depression and insomnia are comorbid and interrelated conditions, and insomnia is often a precursor of, as well as a negative prognostic factor for, depression."

I certainly don't in any way mean to underestimate the potential seriousness of postpartum depression, and I would advise any new mother who is feeling depressed to consult with her doctor immediately. But I would also suggest that if your feelings of depression are being fueled by stress and lack of sleep, you need to do whatever you can to get more rest and reduce your stress. I know that's not always easy when there's a new baby in the house, but do go back and reread the tips I provided in chapter 6.

Stress and Emotional Eating

If you're sleep-deprived, stressed, and depressed, you're also more likely to be reaching for energy-dense foods that are high in starch and sugar—what are generally known as comfort foods. The increase in cortisol that naturally accompanies stress leads to emotionally based eating. In addition, when you are stressed, your body mobilizes energy stores by breaking down fat and muscle in order to feed your brain. If you are chronically depressed, you can deplete those energy stores, and eating starchy, energy-dense foods prevents that from happening. The problem is that the combination of increased cortisol output and palatable comfort-food intake increases the storage of calories in abdominal fat.

Another way to avoid emotional eating is to take a few minutes to engage in some stress-reducing activity that doesn't involve putting food in your mouth. A few that I, and many other people, have found most effective are the following:

- **Deep breathing.** This is the kind of breathing that comes all the way from your abdomen. Most of us generally take shallow breaths that come from the chest. And when we're stressed, our breathing becomes even shallower. So when you start to feel overwhelmed, stop what you're doing wherever you are and breathe deeply. As you do that, concentrate on breathing in positive energy and exhaling negative energy. It really works.

- **Yoga.** This brings together mind, body, and spirit. It's slow and gentle, so it doesn't stress the body, and as you mindfully concentrate on each pose, you'll release stress from both your mind and your body. Anyone can do yoga on some level. If you don't have the time or money to take a class, buy or rent a DVD and do it right in your own living room while your baby looks on—or is napping.

- **Tai chi.** This is a kind of meditation in action. It combines mental concentration, slow breathing, and dance-type movements that flow into one another. Studies have shown that it can significantly reduce resting blood pressure and perceived stress. Again, if you can't get to a class, you can buy or rent a DVD and learn it on you own.

- **Walking meditation.** In a minute we'll talk about the many benefits of brisk walking, but walking meditation is something different. Whereas in seated meditation you generally try to clear your mind and focus on your breathing, in walking meditation you become mindful of the physical sensations involved in each step: your foot hitting the ground, your breathing, the sensation of the sun or the wind on your face. You don't have to do it for very long—just the time it takes you to walk from your house to your car or the bus. You'll be amazed at how quickly your feelings of stress are reduced.

- **A personal mantra.** Create a phrase to repeat to yourself whenever you feel stress coming on. What always works for me is mentally repeating "Trust in God" for ten seconds. You should use whatever works for you.

Also, listen to music, unclutter your schedule and your life, enjoy the beauty of nature, embrace your family and friends, attend religious services (numerous studies have shown the effectiveness of attending religious services of any kind), and don't underestimate the power of prayer.

WHEN YOU'RE STRESSED, EAT TURKEY

You know how sleepy you feel after Thanksgiving dinner? It's not just because you ate too much. It's because turkey is full of tryptophan, an essential amino acid and a precursor to the neurotransmitter serotonin, which is important for mood regulation. Elevated levels of serotonin help us to cope with stress and alleviate depression. So if you're stressed, instead of eating energy-dense comfort foods, reach for one of the following, all of which are rich in tryptophan:

- Skinless turkey or chicken breast
- Wild Alaskan salmon
- Soy beans
- Sardines
- Pumpkin seeds

The Many Benefits of Physical Activity

Our Paleolithic ancestors burned approximately 1,000 calories a day in physical activity, whereas we now burn about 300 while we consume more and more calories every year. If you eat 100 calories more than you burn off as energy every day, in one year you'll have gained ten pounds. That's why physical activity is so important for weight control, but it's important for other reasons as well.

The Mayo Clinic says the following:

> Virtually any form of exercise, from aerobics to weightlifting, can act as a stress reliever. If you're not an athlete or even if you're downright out of shape, you can still make a little exercise go a long way toward stress management. . . . Regular exercise can increase self-confidence and lower the symptoms associated with mild depression and anxiety. Exercise also can improve your sleep, which is often disrupted by stress, depression, and anxiety. All this can ease your stress levels and give you a sense of command over your body and your life.

The Cleveland Clinic concurs. "Regular aerobic exercise can help relieve mild to moderate degrees of depression and anxiety. People who exercise also have less loneliness and anger and are better able to control their own destiny. It is not clear whether exercise boosts the immune system directly or works through a link with the brain and nervous system."

We all know that exercise is good for cardiovascular fitness, but because it reduces stress, which can suppress the immune system, physical activity will also help to ward off a host of opportunistic illnesses.

For all of these reasons, and also, of course, to lose the weight gained during pregnancy and avoid gaining more, physical activity is extremely important in the postpartum period. Unfortunately, studies have found that most women do not receive enough information about lifestyle behaviors and activities from their health-care provider, and one of the reasons many women do not resume physical activity after pregnancy is that they lack information about how to go about it. But now you won't have that excuse!

The *2008 Physical Activity Guidelines for Americans* published by the U.S. Department of Health and Human Services recommends two and a half hours, or 150 minutes, of moderate-intensity aerobic activity spread over the course of a week for postpartum women who are healthy but not already highly active. To determine when and at what level to start your own exercise program, talk to your health-care provider.

Probably the easiest way to start getting active is to simply get out and walk. Walking has been shown to increase HDL (good) cholesterol and lower LDL (bad) cholesterol. Slow walking outdoors, in a country or forest setting (or in a park, if you live in an urban environment), is the most effective way to lose weight and keep it off. In addition, walking outside in nature has been shown to lower pulse rate and blood pressure. It increases activity in your parasympathetic nervous system (the "chilling out" part of your brain) and decreases activity in your sympathetic nervous system (what goes into high gear when you're in fight-or-flight mode). It improves your mood and lowers cortisol levels, which will lessen your comfort food cravings.

Almost anyone can walk. We all learned how a long time ago, and the only necessary equipment is a good pair of shoes and appropriate, comfortable clothing. Assuming that the weather isn't too hot or too cold, you can put your baby in the stroller and walk together. You may find that both of you will sleep better. Access the websites listed in chapter 6, purchase a pedometer, and get moving!

Where You Are Now

If you've been following my guidelines, your baby is on the way to enjoying a long, healthy life. You're protecting him or her, to the best of your ability, from most of the chronic diseases and conditions that are so prevalent in modern society. At the same time, you're protecting yourself from those diseases and conditions. You're at a point where your infant is about to become a toddler who will begin to eat complementary foods and start exploring more of the immediate world on his or her own.

To take you any further on the parenthood path would be to start a whole new book, so this seems like a logical place for me to leave you—confident in your ability to keep on doing everything you've been doing, starting with preconception and continuing through pregnancy and breast-feeding, so that you continue to guide your healthy baby through a healthy childhood and enjoy a healthy life yourself.

I'd also like to point out that most of the environmental, lifestyle, and nutritional choices you've found in this book are truly harking back to an earlier time when virtually all babies were breast-fed, our diets consisted primarily of whole, home-cooked foods, and we didn't have all the chemicals that have become part of modern life. It seems that just a few short generations back, we were living much closer to the way our ancestors did—and for which we are genetically programmed.

For every safety measure we've introduced to protect our children—from bike helmets to car seats—we've also created far more life-threatening possibilities introduced in the name of "progress." So my advice would be this: try doing things the old-fashioned way!

A book I've found to be helpful for dealing with family concerns not related to the issues discussed here is *For Better: 30 Days of Building a Better Family* by Bob Botsford.

PART 4

Recipes, Shopping List, and Supplements

In chapter 10 I'll share some of my family's favorite SuperFoods recipes. I hope that you enjoy them and that they'll inspire you to create new ones of your own. If so, I'd be happy to have you share them with me at http://www.superfoodsrx.com/pregnancybook.

In chapter 11 I'll provide you with a list of products (in addition to those I've already mentioned throughout the text) that I've found to be both tasty and healthy, along with information about where you can find them. Finally, in chapter 12, I'll suggest specific supplements that I believe to be most useful for most people.

I hope that all of these recipes and suggestions will help you as you embark on a superhealthy pregnancy and parenthood.

10

Dr. Steve's Favorite Recipes

Most of these recipes are not created by professional chefs, and they certainly don't require a great deal of skill to prepare. They're the dishes my wife and I, our children, and our friends use on a daily basis, and I want to thank all who were generous enough to let us include their favorites. The number of servings provided is the one that works for us; you may find that they serve more or fewer people, depending on the appetites of your own family members and friends. This is not a "diet" book, and so there are no restrictions on portion sizes or calories. In any case, if you consume a diet comprised mainly of SuperFoods you will, as I've said, lose weight naturally as you also maximize your health.

Quick and Easy SuperFoods Recipes

• •

Kale Omelet
MAKES 2 SERVINGS

Get tasty doses of all of the necessary food groups in this delicious omelet.

6 medium eggs (preferably free-range organic)
¼ cup soy milk
2 tablespoons extra-virgin olive oil, plus additional for greasing the omelet pan
1 cup chopped kale
1 orange bell pepper, diced
½ onion, chopped
1 cup shredded mozzarella cheese

In a small bowl, beat the eggs with the soy milk and set aside.

Heat the 2 tablespoons of olive oil in a medium frying pan. Add the kale, bell pepper, and onion and sauté until soft, about 10 minutes.

Grease the bottom of a small frying pan with olive oil, add half of the egg mixture, and cook over low heat just until it sets. Spread half of the sautéed vegetables over the eggs, and sprinkle with half of the cheese. Fold the omelet in half and serve.

Repeat with the remaining ingredients for a second omelet.

• •

Pumpkin Pancakes
MAKES 6 TO 8 PANCAKES

Pumpkin is so nutritious that it makes pancakes a health food!

1½ cups soy milk

1 15-ounce can pumpkin puree

1 egg (preferably free-range organic)

2 tablespoons distilled white vinegar

2 tablespoons grapeseed oil

¼ cup honey

1¾ cups whole-wheat flour

¼ cup flaxseed

2 teaspoons baking powder

1 teaspoon baking soda

1 teaspoon ground allspice

1 teaspoon ground cinnamon

½ teaspoon ground ginger

extra-virgin olive oil cooking spray or Smart Balance
     Organic Whipped Buttery Spread for the pan

Combine the soy milk, pumpkin, egg, vinegar, oil, and honey in a large bowl.

In a separate bowl, combine the flour, flaxseed, baking powder, baking soda, and spices.

Pour the dry mixture into the pumpkin mixture and stir to combine.

Grease a pancake griddle with the cooking spray or Smart Balance and heat. Ladle a small portion of the pancake mixture onto the hot griddle. Cook until the bottom is just browned, flip, and brown the other side. Repeat with the remaining pancake mixture, adding more cooking spray or Smart Balance to the griddle as necessary.

• •

Bridie's Granola

MAKES 10 SERVINGS

Bridie is my personal trainer, and I thank her not only for her good work but also for allowing me to use her recipe in my book.

3 cups rolled oats

½ cup oat bran

½ cup wheat germ

1 cup walnut pieces

¾ cup sliced almonds

½ cup pumpkin seeds

¼ cup chia seeds

¼ cup dried cranberries

¼ cup currants

½ cup brown sugar

¼ cup agave

¼ cup dark honey

¼ cup almond butter

1 tablespoon water

1 tablespoon vanilla extract

1 tablespoon extra-virgin olive oil

1 tablespoon ground cinnamon

1 teaspoon ground cardamom

½ teaspoon salt

In a large bowl, combine the oats, bran, wheat germ, nuts, seeds, cranberries, and currants. Set aside.

Preheat the oven to 325 degrees.

Combine all of the remaining ingredients in a medium saucepan and stir over medium heat for 3 minutes.

Stir the sweet mixture into the dry mixture and transfer the granola to a 15 × 10 inch jelly roll pan. Bake for 30 minutes.

Remove from the oven and cool for 15 minutes before serving.

Store leftovers in the pantry or cupboard for up to one week in a lidded glass container.

• •

. . . .

Guni's Tortilla Soup

MAKES 4 SERVINGS

This is my wife's recipe. It's filling and delicious. Have a bowl for lunch or a light dinner.

- 2 tablespoons extra-virgin olive oil
- 1 large onion, chopped
- 1 cup diced orange bell pepper
- ¼ cup chopped fresh cilantro
- 4 cups low-sodium chicken broth
- 2 chicken breasts, cooked and chopped into bite-size pieces
- 2 teaspoons minced garlic
- 2 teaspoons dried oregano
- 1 28-ounce can diced tomatoes with liquid
- 2 teaspoons ground cumin
- ½ teaspoon dried thyme
- ½ teaspoon freshly ground black pepper
- 4 cups broken-up yellow corn tortilla chips
- 1 avocado, chopped

Heat the olive oil in a skillet over medium heat. Add the onion, bell pepper, and cilantro, and cook, stirring, until the onion is soft.

Transfer to a large pot and add the broth, chicken, garlic, oregano, tomatoes, cumin, thyme, and pepper. Cover, reduce the heat, and simmer for 1 hour.

Divide the tortilla chips among 4 bowls. Ladle the soup over the chips and garnish with the avocado.

. . . .

• •

Janice's Baja Butternut Soup
MAKES 6 SERVINGS

Janice Hart Rooney is a friend and a food blogger who has kindly allowed me to use her healthy and delicious recipe.

   1½ pounds (1 small or medium) butternut or other winter squash
   1 teaspoon canola oil
   2 stalks celery, chopped
   1 small onion, diced
   1 carrot, chopped
   1 teaspoon ground cumin
   ¼ to ½ teaspoon chipotle chili powder
   ⅛ teaspoon ground cloves
   6 cups vegetable broth
   2 ears corn, husked
   1 teaspoon sea salt
   ¼ teaspoon freshly ground black pepper
   chopped fresh chives or flat-leaf parsley, for garnish

Preheat the oven to 350 degrees.

Cut the squash in half and seed it. Place the halves on a baking sheet, cut side down, and bake until tender when pierced with a knife, 45 minutes to 1 hour. When cool enough to handle, scoop out the flesh.

Heat the oil in a large saucepan over medium heat. Add the celery, onion, and carrot and stir to coat. Cover, reduce the heat to medium-low, and cook, stirring frequently, until soft, 8 to 10 minutes. Stir in the squash flesh, cumin, chipotle powder to taste, and cloves. Add the broth and simmer, covered, until the vegetables are very tender, 20 to 25 minutes.

Meanwhile, heat the grill (or a grill pan) to medium heat and grill the corn, turning occasionally, until lightly grilled but not charred. Slice the kernels off the cobs.

Puree the soup with an immersion blender or in a regular blender (in batches) until smooth. (Use caution when pureeing hot liquids.) Add the corn kernels, season with salt and pepper, and garnish with the chopped chives or parsley.

• •

Grant's Guacamole
MAKES 6 APPETIZER-SIZE SERVINGS

Avocados have all kinds of healthy nutrients. Enjoy your guacamole with some of the chips listed in chapter 11 or, as my son Grant suggests, with Torey's Kale Chips (next recipe).

4 avocados
1 tablespoon chili powder
1 tablespoon taco sauce (I prefer La Victoria)
½ teaspoon fresh lemon juice

Peel the avocados and mash them in a large bowl.

Stir in the remaining ingredients. Cover airtight and refrigerate for 30 minutes.

Serve immediately.

• •

Torey's Kale Chips
MAKES 2 TO 4 SERVINGS

This is my daughter's recipe. She says they make a great appetizer or snack, and she's right. Kale is also full of nutrients and antioxidants.

1 tablespoon extra-virgin olive oil
½ teaspoon salt (optional)
2 teaspoons crushed garlic
6 cups chopped fresh kale (bite-size pieces)

Preheat the oven to 350 degrees.

Combine the olive oil, salt, and garlic in a small bowl.

Put the kale pieces in large bowl and pour the olive oil mixture on top. Toss like a salad until all of the kale is covered with the oil mixture.

Spread the kale evenly on a large cookie sheet and bake until crisp, about 10 minutes. Turn the chips over and bake 5 more minutes.

• •

SuperFoods Spinach Salad
MAKES 2 SERVINGS

This salad is full of all kinds of good things, and it tastes great, too.

Salad
1 cup chopped spinach (bite-size pieces)
1 cup chopped romaine lettuce
¼ cup shredded red cabbage
½ cup sliced red, orange, or yellow bell pepper
½ cup chopped tomato
¼ cup canned chickpeas, drained and rinsed well
½ cup grated carrot
¼ avocado, cubed

Dressing
2 tablespoons extra-virgin olive oil
1 teaspoon balsamic vinegar

Optional Garnishes
freshly ground pepper to taste
chopped fresh herbs of your choice
1 tablespoon freshly grated Parmesan cheese
2 tablespoons roasted nuts or seeds

Combine the spinach, romaine lettuce, cabbage, pepper, tomato, chickpeas, carrot, and avocado in a large bowl.

In a separate bowl, combine the oil and vinegar.

Toss the dressing with the salad just before serving. If you like, add the garnishes of your choice.

• •

Corn Salad
MAKES 4 SERVINGS

This is a great side dish to serve at a barbecue.

Salad
1 15-ounce can corn niblets
1 15-ounce can black beans
1 orange bell pepper, diced
1 red bell pepper, diced
1 zucchini, diced
1 small onion, diced
3 stalks celery, chopped

Dressing
3 tablespoons fresh lemon juice
3 tablespoons extra-virgin olive oil
1 teaspoon freshly ground black pepper

Combine all of the salad ingredients in a medium bowl.

Combine the dressing ingredients in a small bowl.

Toss the salad with the dressing and serve.

• •

● ●

Herb-Crusted Salmon Salad

MAKES 2 TO 4 SERVINGS

This recipe is from *Racing to the Table: A Culinary Tour of Racing America* by Margaret Guthrie.

Salad

2 tablespoons raspberry vinegar

½ cup extra-virgin olive oil

½ teaspoon honey

1 teaspoon finely minced garlic

salt and freshly ground black pepper to taste

4 cups shredded baby lettuce leaves

Herb Mixture

1½ cups panko bread crumbs

½ cup freshly grated Parmesan cheese

¼ cup chopped fresh basil

¼ cup chopped fresh flat-leaf parsley

2 tablespoons dried oregano

2 tablespoons dried thyme

1 tablespoon garlic powder

Salmon

6 ounces wild Atlantic salmon fillets

freshly ground black pepper to taste

4 tablespoons Dijon mustard

2 to 4 tablespoons (¼ to ½ stick) organic butter

In a small bowl combine the vinegar, olive oil, honey, garlic, salt, and pepper and whisk well to emulsify. Toss with the baby lettuce and set aside.

In a wide, shallow bowl, combine the bread crumbs with the grated cheese, herbs, and garlic powder and mix well to blend completely. Set aside.

Preheat the oven to 425 degrees.

Sprinkle the salmon with the pepper and spread the mustard evenly on top. Press the mustard-covered salmon into the bread crumb mixture and set aside.

Heat the butter in a large, heavy-bottomed, ovenproof sauté pan over medium heat. Add the salmon and brown for 2 to 3 minutes.

Transfer the pan to the preheated oven and bake for about 15 minutes. Watch the fish carefully, because the cooking time will depend on the thickness of the fillets.

Spread the dressed greens on a platter, top with the salmon, and serve.

• •

Broiled Wild Alaskan Salmon

MAKES 2 TO 4 SERVINGS

Wild Alaskan salmon is one of my favorite SuperFoods, and this is one of my favorite salmon recipes. The honey is good for you, too!

¼ cup extra-virgin olive oil

¼ cup honey

2 tablespoons minced fresh rosemary

2 tablespoons fresh lemon juice

1 pound wild Alaskan salmon fillets

In a small bowl (we use glass because it is a nontoxic material), combine the olive oil, honey, rosemary, and lemon juice and mix well.

Place the salmon fillets in a baking dish large enough to hold them in a single layer and pour the sauce over the top.

Heat the broiler and broil the salmon until the top is opaque and the fish flakes easily with a fork, 10 to 15 minutes, depending on the thickness of the fillets.

• •

• •

Sweet Salsa Salmon
MAKES 2 TO 4 SERVINGS

The tangy, fruity salsa gives this salmon dish extra zing.

Salsa
1 ripe mango, peeled and diced
1 15-ounce can crushed pineapple, drained
1 tomato, diced
1 small onion, diced
½ cup chopped fresh cilantro
1 teaspoon fresh lemon juice

Salmon
1 pound wild Alaskan salmon fillets
2 tablespoons olive oil
freshly ground black pepper to taste

Preheat the oven to 400 degrees.

Combine the salsa ingredients in a bowl and set aside.

Place the salmon in a baking dish large enough to hold the fillets in a single layer. Prick with a fork several times. Spread the olive oil on top and sprinkle with the pepper to taste.

Bake until the fish is opaque on top and flakes easily with a fork, 10 to 15 minutes, depending on the thickness of the fillets.

Remove from the oven, top with the salsa, and serve.

• •

Mike's "Deluxe" Bean Dish
MAKES 2 TO 4 SERVINGS

This is my son's creation. Nothing could be easier!

1 15-ounce can black beans

1 15-ounce can Health Valley vegetarian chili, no salt added

1 tablespoon wheat bran

1 tablespoon extra-virgin olive oil

1 teaspoon onion powder

1 teaspoon garlic powder

1 teaspoon dried basil

1 teaspoon dried oregano

2 teaspoons honey

½ cup diced orange bell pepper or carrot

¼ teaspoon freshly ground black pepper

½ cup shredded cheese of your choice

In a medium-size glass pan, combine all the ingredients except the cheese. Sprinkle the cheese over the bean mixture, cover the pan with a paper towel or wax paper, and microwave for 3 to 4 minutes or until hot.

• •

Black Bean Turkey Chili

MAKES 4 TO 6 SERVINGS

Black beans and turkey make chili a SuperFood, so don't be afraid to indulge.

2 tablespoons extra-virgin olive oil

1 pound ground turkey

1 medium onion, diced

2 tomatoes, diced

2 30-ounce cans black beans, with liquid

½ cup chili powder

2 teaspoons minced garlic

2 teaspoons ground cumin

2 6-ounce cans tomato paste

1 cup water

1 14½-ounce can tomato sauce

¼ cup honey
½ cup ketchup
1 teaspoon freshly ground black pepper

Heat the oil in a pan large enough to hold all of the ingredients. Add the turkey and brown, stirring frequently, until all the pink is gone.

Add the onion and cook, stirring often, until soft, about 5 minutes.

Add all of the remaining ingredients, combine thoroughly, and simmer, stirring, until hot.

• •

Turkey Meat Loaf

MAKES 4 SERVINGS

Everyone loves meat loaf, and this turkey version is full of antioxidant-rich vegetables.

2 tablespoons extra-virgin olive oil
1 medium onion, diced
½ cup diced orange bell pepper
½ cup diced red bell pepper
¼ cup diced celery
1 teaspoon dried oregano
½ teaspoon freshly ground black pepper
1 egg (preferably free-range organic)
1 pound ground turkey
1 6-oz can tomato paste
½ cup whole-wheat bread crumbs
1 tablespoon ground flaxseed
cooking spray
1 tablespoon ketchup

Preheat the oven to 350 degrees.

In a medium frying pan, heat the olive oil over medium heat. Add the onion, red and orange bell peppers, celery, oregano, and black pepper. Sauté until the onion is slightly browned, 3 to 4 minutes.

In a large bowl, lightly beat the egg. Add the ground turkey and mix well. (It's okay to use your hands.) Add the sautéed vegetables and the tomato paste, bread crumbs, and flaxseed, and mix well.

Spray a loaf pan with cooking spray and transfer the turkey mixture to the pan, pressing it down evenly. Spread the ketchup over the top and cover with foil. Bake for 45 minutes.

Let the meat loaf sit for a few minutes before you slice it.

• •

Turkey Fried Brown Rice

MAKES 2 MAIN-DISH SERVINGS OR 4 SIDE-DISH SERVINGS

Stay away from fried rice in Chinese restaurants and enjoy this one instead. It can be either a main dish or a side dish served with salmon.

    3 tablespoons extra-virgin olive oil
    1 cup chopped onion
    2 tomatoes, chopped
    2 cups chopped fresh spinach
    2 cups chopped cooked turkey breast
    3 cups cooked brown rice
    1 teaspoon freshly ground black pepper
    2 tablespoons minced garlic
    1 teaspoon paprika
    3 eggs, scrambled (preferably free-range organic)

Heat the olive oil in a large frying pan. Add the onion and sauté, stirring frequently, until just beginning to brown.

Add the tomatoes and spinach and cook for about 5 minutes, until the vegetables are soft.

Add all of the remaining ingredients and fry on medium heat, stirring, until heated through.

• •

Macaroni Bake

MAKES 6 TO 8 SERVINGS

Is there anyone on earth who doesn't love macaroni? If so, I haven't met them yet!

 3 tablespoons extra-virgin olive oil, plus additional for greasing the pan
 1 pound ground turkey
 1 large onion, diced
 2 tomatoes, chopped
 2 6-ounce cans tomato paste
 1 tablespoon dried oregano
 1 tablespoon dried basil
 1 tablespoon crushed dried bay leaf
 1 teaspoon dried thyme
 1 teaspoon freshly ground black pepper
 4 cups cooked whole-wheat elbow macaroni
 2 cups shredded cheese of your choice

Heat the 3 tablespoons of olive oil in a large frying pan. Add the turkey and sauté over medium heat, stirring frequently, until browned.

Add the onion and chopped tomatoes and cook, stirring, for about 10 minutes, until soft.

Add all of the remaining ingredients except the macaroni and cheese and simmer for 30 minutes.

Preheat the oven to 400 degrees.

Off the heat, combine the tomato mixture with the maca- roni and transfer to a baking dish greased with olive oil. Sprinkle with the cheese, cover with foil, and bake for 30 minutes.

• •

Easy Black Bean Brownies
MAKES 4 2-SQUARE-INCH BROWNIES

Serve these, and people will ask for the recipe. Then they won't believe you when you tell them.

    1 15-ounce can black beans, drained
    3 large eggs (preferably free-range organic)
    3 tablespoons canola oil
    ¾ cup sugar
    ½ cup ground pure cocoa powder
    1½ teaspoons vanilla
    ½ teaspoon baking powder
    ½ cup chopped dark chocolate (70 percent cocoa or
      higher)
    cooking spray

Preheat the oven to 350 degrees.

Place the black beans in a blender or a food proces- sor and blend until creamy. Add the eggs, oil, sugar, cocoa powder, vanilla and baking powder and blend. Add the chopped chocolate and blend just until combined.

Coat an 8 × 8 inch baking pan with nonstick cooking spray. Spread the batter in the pan and bake for 30 to 35 minutes, until the brownies spring back when pressed with your finger.

Remove from the oven and let them cool in the pan. When they are cool, cut them into squares.

• •

Guni's Oatmeal, Honey, and Pumpkin Cookies

MAKES 2 DOZEN COOKIES

These are great with your favorite organic jam.

½ cup (1 stick) organic butter, softened
½ cup honey
1½ cups canned pumpkin
1 egg (preferably free-range organic)
1 teaspoon vanilla extract
2 cups whole-wheat flour
1 teaspoon baking powder
1 teaspoon baking soda
1 tablespoon ground cinnamon
1 teaspoon ground allspice
1 cup rolled oats
cooking spray

Preheat the oven to 350 degrees.

In a large bowl, mix the butter and honey. Blend in the pumpkin, then add the egg and vanilla.

In a second bowl, combine all of the remaining ingredients (except the cooking spray).

Slowly mix the dry ingredients into the pumpkin mixture.

Spray a cookie sheet with the cooking spray and drop rounded teaspoons of the batter onto the pan, about an inch apart. Bake for 11 to 12 minutes.

Remove and serve warm or cold.

• •

• •

Florence Quinn's Beet Muffins
MAKES 6 MEDIUM-SIZE MUFFINS

Florence Quinn is a professional chef and a clinical nutritionist who cooks with fresh, local, unprocessed foods. I'm grateful to her for permission to use this recipe. These muffins are loaded with nutrients and good fats and contain little added sugar.

1 medium (or 3 small) red beet(s), unpeeled
drizzle of extra-virgin olive oil
pinch of salt and freshly ground black pepper
a little water
½ cup unsweetened coconut milk
1 teaspoon fresh lemon juice
1 egg (preferably free-range organic)
¼ cup natural brown cane sugar
¼ cup extra-virgin olive oil
¾ cup all-purpose flour
½ cup almond flour
1 tablespoon chia seeds or poppy seeds
¾ teaspoon baking powder
¼ teaspoon baking soda
¼ teaspoon sea salt

Preheat the oven to 400 degrees.

Place the unpeeled beet(s) in a baking dish, add the drizzle of olive oil and the pinch of salt and pepper, and toss the beet(s) to lightly coat with oil. Add enough water to cover the bottom of the pan by ½ inch.

Cover with foil, and with a sharp knife, make a few small incisions in the foil to allow the steam to escape.

Roast for 45 to 70 minutes, depending on the size of the beet(s), until very soft. Remove from the oven and allow to cool before peeling. (Use your fingers; the skin will slip right off.)

Puree in a food processor until smooth. Reserve ¼ cup of the puree for the muffins; you can freeze any leftover puree for another time.

Reduce the oven to 350 degrees.

In a medium bowl, whisk the ¼ cup of pureed beets with the coconut milk, lemon juice, egg, sugar, and ¼ cup of olive oil until just combined. Set aside.

In a large bowl, combine the flours, seeds, baking powder and soda, and sea salt.

Add the wet ingredients to the dry ingredients and whisk to combine.

Line 6 muffin cups with baking paper and spoon the batter into the lined cups. Bake in the preheated oven for 22 minutes or until a fork inserted in the center of a muffin comes out clean. Cool on a rack.

These muffins are best eaten on the day they are made.

• •

Butternut Squash Cake with Coconut, Cranberries, and Walnuts

MAKES 1 10-INCH LOAF

Here's another great recipe from Florence Quinn. The squash and coconut provide natural sweetness, so there is little sugar added.

    cooking spray
    1 cup whole-wheat flour
    ½ cup all-purpose flour
    1 teaspoon baking soda
    ½ cup fine-grain natural cane sugar or brown sugar
    1 teaspoon salt
    2 eggs (preferably free-range organic)

¾ cup pureed roasted butternut squash

6 tablespoons unsweetened coconut milk

6 tablespoons extra-virgin olive oil

2 tablespoons honey

2 tablespoons finely grated peeled ginger root

finely grated zest of 1 lemon

½ cup coarsely chopped toasted walnuts or pecans

½ cup dried cranberries or sour cherries (no sugar added)

Preheat the oven to 375 degrees.

Spray a 10-inch loaf pan with cooking spray. Combine the flours, baking soda, sugar, and salt in a large bowl and set aside.

In a food processor, blend the eggs, squash, coconut milk, olive oil, honey, ginger, and lemon zest until smooth. Add to the flour mixture, and stir until just combined. Fold in the nuts and dried berries.

Pour the batter into the prepared pan and bake for about 1 hour, until the edges have browned and a fork inserted in the center of the cake comes out clean.

Allow to cool in the pan. Eat this cake in the next two days, or freeze individual slices for delayed enjoyment.

• •

Good-for-You Chocolate Milk (Hot or Cold)

MAKES 1 SERVING

As I noted in an earlier chapter, dark chocolate is actually a health food!

8 ounces soy milk

1 scoop whey protein powder

1 tablespoon pure cocoa powder

1 tablespoon honey

Pour the soy milk into a large glass or mug. Stir in the protein powder, then the cocoa powder and honey. Drink it cold or heat in the microwave for hot chocolate.

Recipes for Natural Beauty

My friend Shari White worked for many years in the skin-care department of Elizabeth Arden. I am grateful to her for allowing me to share these green beauty recipes with you.

• •

Apple-Honey Mask for Acne-Prone Skin

The grains of apple work as a sort of gentle exfoliator, cleaning the dead skin from your face. The glycolic acid becomes a natural facial scrub, penetrating deep into the pores. The honey is nature's antioxidant and has antimicrobial properties that alleviate the problems that cause acne. It works best when made fresh for each application, but you can make it a few days in advance and refrigerate it until you're ready to use it.

1 apple
warm honey

Peel and core the apple. Put the flesh in a blender or use a handheld electric mixer to mash it into pulp. Add the warm honey and keep blending until you have a fine paste.

Using two fingers, cover your entire face with a layer of the apple-honey paste. You can also apply it to your neck and upper chest, if you wish. Then relax for 10 to 15 minutes to allow the mask to dry. Remove it with a soft washcloth and some warm water.

• •

Nature's Moisturizer for Dry Skin

Just open a jar of honey and smooth it onto your face once a week. Before applying, warm the honey in the microwave and moisten your skin with warm water. Leave the honey on for 30 minutes and remove with a soft washcloth and some warm water. The honey not only nourishes your skin but also leaves it soft, smooth, and supple.

• •

Banana-Honey Oatmeal Face Mask for Sensitive Skin

I love the way this face mask smells. It is good for all skin types, but especially great for sensitive skin. Oatmeal is high in nourishing vitamins and minerals; it gently cleanses and heals skin. Bananas contain vitamin A, which helps to moisturize and soothe the skin. Honey helps to maintain the skin's natural acid mantle.

¼ cup oatmeal

¼ cup milk or yogurt

½ tablespoon honey

½ banana, mashed

1 egg (preferably free-range organic)

Mix the oatmeal with the milk or yogurt, then combine with the rest of the ingredients and warm in the microwave. Use your fingers to gently massage the mask onto the skin in slow circular motions. Wait about 15 minutes, then rinse with warm water.

• •

• •

Hot Honey Hair Mask

Give your hair and scalp a great treatment using nature's best. Organic honey and olive oil combine to make a fabulous conditioner. This hair mask will leave you with soft, smooth, frizz-free, shiny hair that looks as if you'd just had an expensive salon treatment.

½ cup honey
½ cup olive oil

Combine the honey and the olive oil and warm the mixture in the microwave. Starting at the roots of your hair and working toward the ends, apply to clean, towel-dried but still damp hair.

Wrap your hair up in a towel and wait 20 minutes. Shampoo again and dry your hair as usual.

• •

11

Your SuperFoods Shopping List

This chapter lists some of my favorite SuperFoods products. I've indicated throughout which ones are organic. Not every one of them will be available in every market or in every part of the country, but you can check the manufacturer's website or call for availability by mail or in your area. You can also find your own local brands based on the ingredients that are in the products listed below. Most large supermarket chains, including Walmart and Costco, now have an organic produce section.

Foods and Beverages

Applesauce

Santa Cruz Organic Cinnamon Apple Sauce, http://www.santa cruzorganic.com

Trader Joe's Organic Apple Sauce, unsweetened, http://www
.traderjoes.com

Bread
Organic

Alpine Valley Organic Sprouted Honey Wheat with Flaxseed,
1-480-483-2774

Food for Life: The Original Flourless Sprouted Grain Bread
Ezekiel 4:9, low sodium, http://www.foodforlife.com

Food for Life: The Original Flourless Sprouted Grain Burger
Buns Ezekiel 4:9, Sesame, http://www.foodforlife.com

Julian Bakery Low Carb Smart Carb #1 Bread (a complete
sprouted high-protein bread), http://www.julianbakery.com

Julian Bakery Oat Bran (a complete protein bread), http://
www.julianbakery.com

Julian Bakery Bible Recipe (a complete protein bread),
http://www.julianbakery.com

Rudi's Organic Bakery 7 Grain with Flax Bread, http://www
.rudisbakery.com

Rudi's Organic Bakery Cinnamon Raisin Bagels, http://
www.rudisbakery.com

Nonorganic

Sara Lee Healthy Multi-Grain Bread, http://www.saralee
.com

Cereal
Organic

365 Organic Chia Seed, http://www.wholefoodsmarket.com

365 Organic Multi Grain with Flax Instant Oatmeal (hot
cereal), http://www.wholefoodsmarket.com

Arrowhead Mills Organic Oat Bran Hot Cereal, http://www
.arrowheadmills.com

Arrowhead Mills Organic Sprouted Multigrain Flakes,
http://www.arrowheadmills.com

Bob's Red Mill Organic Whole Grain Steel Cut Oats (hot cereal), http://www.bobsredmill.com

Bob's Red Mill Organic Whole Ground Flaxseed Meal, http://www.bobsredmill.com

Food for Life Ezekiel 4:9 Cinnamon Raisin (a sprouted whole-grain cereal), http://www.foodforlife.com

Food for Life Ezekiel 4:9 Golden Flax (a sprouted whole-grain cereal), http://www.foodforlife.com

Food for Life Ezekiel 4:9 Original (a sprouted whole-grain cereal), http://www.foodforlife.com

Nature's Path 3 Generations Organic Flax Plus Raisin Bran, http://www.naturespath.com

Nature's Path 3 Generations Organic Flax Plus Multibran Flakes, http://www.naturespath.com

Nature's Path 3 Generations Organic Flax Plus Pumpkin Raisin Crunch, http://www.naturespath.com

Nature's Path 3 Generations Organic Heritage Flake Ancient Grains, Kamut, http://www.naturespath.com

Nature's Path 3 Generations Organic Multigrain Oatbran Cereal, http://www.naturespath.com

Nature's Path 3 Generations Organic Whole O's, http://www.naturespath.com

Nature's Path Organic Instant Hot Oatmeal Multigrain Raisin Spice, http://www.naturespath.com

Nonorganic

Bob's Red Mill Rice Bran, http://www.bobsredmill.com

Kashi Golean Crunch, http://www.kashi.com

Kashi Golean, http://www.kashi.com

Kashi Honey Sunshine, http://www.kashi.com

Quaker Oat Bran Hot Cereal, http://www.quakeroats.com

Quaker Real Medleys Apple Walnut Oatmeal, http://www.quakeroats.com

Trader Joe's Chia Seeds, http://www.traderjoes.com

Spectrum Chia Seed, http://www.spectrumorganics.com

Trader Joe's Natural Toasted Oat Bran, http://www.traderjoes.com

Chips

Organic

365 Organic Yellow Corn Tortilla Chips or Strips, http://www.wholefoods.com

Kettle Brand Chips (unsalted), http://www.kettlebrand.com

Kettle Brand Krinkle Cut Potato Chips, Organic Roasted Tomato, http://www.kettlebrand.com

Late July Sweet Potato Multigrain Snack Chips, http://www.latejuly.com

Rhythm Superfoods Sweet Potato Chips, Hickory BBQ, http://www.rhythmsuperfoods.com

Nonorganic

Food Should Taste Good Original Sweet Potato Chips, http://www.foodshouldtastegood.com

Food Should Taste Good Barbeque Sweet Potato Chips, http://www.foodshouldtastegood.com

Garden of Eatin' Mini Yellow Rounds, http://www.gardenofeatin.com

Garden of Eatin' Sweet Potato Corn Tortilla Chips (made with organic yellow corn and sweet potato) and other flavors, http://www.gardenofeatin.com

Chocolate, Dark

Cocoa Powder

Dagoba Organic Chocolate Cacao Powder, http://www.dagobachocolate.com/

Rapunzel Organic Cocoa Powder (unsweetened and nonalkaline cocoa for baking and cooking), http://www.rapunzel.com

Candy Bars (Dark Chocolate)

Endangered Species Chocolate All-Natural Extreme Dark Chocolate, 88 percent cocoa (10 percent of net profits donated to help support species, habitat, and humanity), http://www.ChocolateBar.com

Lindt Excellence 85 percent Cocoa Extra Dark, http://www .lindt.com

Vital Choice Organic Chocolate Bars (multiple varieties, all 80 percent cocoa), http://www.vitalchoice.com

Crackers and Crispbreads

Ak-Mak 100% Stone Ground Whole Wheat Sesame Crackers, http://www.akmakbkeries.com

Health Valley Amaranth Graham Crackers, http://www .healthvalley.com

Health Valley Oat Bran Graham Crackers, http://www .healthvalley.com

Health Valley Rice Bran Crackers, http://www.healthvalley .com

Ryvita Dark Rye Whole Grain Crispbread, http://www.ryvita .co.uk/prodoucts/crispbread

Wasa Multi Grain Crispbread, http://www.wasa-usa.com

Fish

Fresh-frozen and available by mail order from http://www .vitalchoice.com

Wild Alaskan Salmon (king, silver, sockeye)

Halibut

Sable fish

Tuna

Shellfish (crab, scallops, shrimp, mussels, clams)

Sardines

Canned

365 Wild Caught Alaskan Red Sockeye Salmon (bones and skin included), http://www.wholefoodsmarket.com

Crown Prince Natural Alaskan Pink Salmon (45 mg of sodium per serving), http://www.crownprince.com

Kirkland Signature Boneless & Skinless Wild Alaskan

Sockeye Salmon, http://www.costco.com

Kirkland Signature Solid White Albacore Tuna (packed in water), http://www.costco.com

Vital Choice BPA-free canned Alaskan salmon, sardines, tuna (also no-sodium-added choices), http://www.vitalchoice .com

Wild Planet Wild Albacore Tuna, http://www.wildplanetfoods .com

Fruit

Dried, Organic

Whole Foods organic goji berries, http://www.wholefoods market.com

Whole Foods organic pitted prunes, http://www.whole foodsmarket.com

Whole Foods organic sour tart cherries, http://www.whole foodsmarket.com

Navitas Pomegranate Powder (freeze dried), http://www .navitasnaturals.com

Goji Berries, http://www.navitasnaturals.com

Dried, Nonorganic

Trader Joe's freeze-dried blueberries, http://www.traderjoes .com

Trader Joe's freeze-dried raspberries, http://www.traderjoes.com

Trader Joe's freeze-dried strawberries, http://www.trader joes.com

Frozen, Organic

Townsend Farms Organic Antioxidant Blend (dark cherries, blueberries, pomegranate arils, red raspberries, and strawberries), http://www.townsendfarms.com

Frozen, Nonorganic*

Trader Joe's Fancy Berry Medley (blueberries, blackberries, and raspberries), http://www.traderjoes.com

Trader Joe's Wild Boreal Blueberries, http://www.traderjoes .com

*Dole and many other companies now package a wide variety of frozen berries and other fruits (and vegetables).

Fruit Juices

Organic

> 365 Organic Honey Crisp Apple Juice, http://www.whole foodsmarket.com
>
> Lakewood Organic Fresh Pressed Pure Black Cherry Juice, http://www.lakewoodjuices.com
>
> Lakewood Organic Fresh Pressed Pure Blueberry Juice, http://www.lakewoodjuices.com
>
> Lakewood Organic Fresh Pressed Pure Concord Grape Juice, http://www.lakewoodjuices.com
>
> Lakewood Organic Pomegranate with Blueberry Juice, http://www.lakewoodjuices.com
>
> R. W. Knudsen Organic Apple Juice, http://www.knudsen juices.com
>
> R. W. Knudsen Organic Prune Juice, http://www.knudsen juices.com
>
> R. W. Knudsen Organic Just Tart Cherry Juice, http://www .knudsenjuices.com
>
> Santa Cruz Organic Concord Grape Juice, http://www .santacruzorganic.com

Nonorganic

> All Natural Nantucket Nectars (multiple flavors), http:// www.juiceguys.com
>
> Kirkland Signature Hansen's Natural 100% Juice (and other varieties), http://www.costco.com
>
> Martinelli's Unfiltered Apple Juice, http://www.martinellis .com
>
> R. W. Knudsen Just Dark Cherry Juice, http://www.knud senjuices.com
>
> TreeTop 100% Apple Juice, http://www.treetop.com
>
> Welch's 100% Concord Grape Juice, http://www.welchs.com

365 Extra Pulp 100% Florida Orange Juice, http://www
.wholefoodsmarket.com

Wyman's Wild Blueberry 100% Juice, http://www.wymans.com

Honey

Look for brands from an area near where you live and
certified for country of origin.

Buckwheat honey, http://www.localharavest.org/
buck-wheat/honey-C5192 or http://www.info.com/
WhereToBuyBuckWheatHoney

Honey Gardens Apitherapy Raw Honey, http://www
.honeygardens.com

Y. S. Organic Bee Farms 100% Certified Organic Raw Honey,
http://www.ysorganic.com

Infant Formula

Similac Advance Organic Complete Nutrition (with Lutein
& DHA), http://www.similac.com

Earth's Best Organic Infant Formula with Iron (with DHA
& ARA), http://www.earthsbest.com

Jam

Bionaturae Organic Bilberry Fruit Spread (and various other
flavors), http://www.bionaturae.com

Legumes

365 Organic Black Beans (and other varieties), http://www
.wholefoodsmarket.com

Westbrae Natural Vegetarian Organic Lentil Beans (and
many other varieties), 1-800-434-4246

Nut Butters

Organic

MaraNatha Organic Roasted Peanut Butter (no added
sodium), http://www.maranathafoods.com

NuttZo Peanut Free Omega-3 Seven Nut & Seed Butter, http:// www.gonuttzo.com

Organic Once Again Crunchy Nut Butter (no salt added), http://www.onceagainnutbutter.com

Organic Once Again 100% Valencia Peanut Butter (no salt added, with skins), http://www.onceagainnutbutter .com

Santa Cruz Organic Peanut Butter, http://www.santacruz organic.com

Nonorganic

Laura Scudders Natural Peanut Butter (no added sodium), http://www.laurascudderspeanutbutter.com/product

MaraNatha Natural Almond Butter (no added sodium), http://www.maranathafoods.com

Nuts and Seeds

Organic

365 Organic Walnuts (halves and pieces), http://www .wholefoodsmarket.com

365 Organic Soynuts Roasted & Salted (40 mg of sodium per $\frac{1}{3}$ cup), http://www.wholefoodsmarket.com

365 Organic Sunflower Kernels Roasted & Unsalted, http:// www.wholefoodsmarket.com

Whole Foods Market Organic Dry Roasted, No Salt Almonds, http://www.wholefoodsmarket.com

Whole Foods Market Organic Dry Roasted, No Salt Whole Cashews, http://www.wholefoodsmarket.com

Vital Choice Organic Walnuts, Almonds, and Cashews, http://www.vitalchoice.com

Nonorganic*

365 Peanuts Roasted & Unsalted, http://www.wholefoods market .com

*Trader Joe's also has a wide variety of raw and dry roasted nuts and seeds, http://www.traderjoes.com.

Olive Oil and Butter Substitutes

100% Organic Colavita Extra-Virgin Olive Oil (first cold-pressed), http://www.colavita.com

Smart Balance Organic Whipped Buttery Spread, http://www.smartbalance.com

Pasta

Organic

Andean Dream Quinoa Pasta (gluten- and corn-free, kosher), http://www.andeandream.com

Lundberg Organic Brown Rice Pasta, http://www.lundberg.com

Organic Whole Wheat Spaghetti, http://www.pandlimports.com

Nonorganic

De Cecco Penne Rigate Whole Wheat Pasta, http://www.dececcousa.com

Pumpkin

Libby's 100% Pure Pumpkin, http://www.VeryBestBaking.com

Stonewall Kitchen Maple Pumpkin Butter, 1-800-207-JAMS

Salad Greens

Fresh Express, http://www.freshexpress.com

Mann's, http://www.veggiesmadeeasy.com

Cut'n Clean Greens, http://www.cutnclean.com

Sodas

Reed's All Natural Jamaican Style Ginger Ale, http://www.REEDSGingerBrew.com

Soups

Health Valley Organic No Salt Added Black Bean Soup, http://www.healthvalley.com

Health Valley Organic No Salt Added Lentil Soup, http://
www.healthvalley.com

Trader Joe's Organic Butternut Squash Soup (low sodium),
http://www.traderjoes.com

Trader Joe's Organic Tomato & Roasted Red Pepper Soup
(low sodium), http://www.traderjoes.com

Soy Milk

Organic

365 Organic Soymilk (various flavors), http://www.whole
foodsmarket.com

Kirkland Signature Organic Soymilk (various flavors),
http://www.costco.com

Silk soymilk (various flavors), http://www.silk.com

Nonorganic

Silk All Natural Soymilk (various flavors), http://www
.silk.com

Spices

Organic

Kirkland Signature Organic No Salt Seasoning (one of my
all-time favorite products), http://www.costco.com

McCormick Gourmet Collection herbs and spices (various),
http://www.mccormickgourmet.com

Vital Choice organic spices (many varieties), http://www
.vitalchoice.com

Nonorganic

Mrs. Dash Seasoning Blend (salt-free, various flavors),
http://www.mrsdash.com

Kirkland Signature Tellicherry Black Pepper Grinder, http://
www.costco.com

Rosanna's Pasta Italian Seasoning (basil, oregano, and rosemary), http://www.rosannaspastashop.com

Vegetable Juices

Columbia Gorge Organic Pure Pressed Carrot Juice, http://www.cogojuice.com

Kirkland Signature Bolthouse Farms Organic 100% Carrot Juice, http://www.costco.com

R. W. Knudsen Organic Orange Carrot Juice, http://www.knudsenjuices.com

R. W. Knudsen Very Veggie Juice (organic, low-sodium), http://www.knudsenjuices.com

Vinegar

Stump's Family Marketplace aged balsamic vinegar, 1-858-277-6192

Water, Bottled in Plastic

Glaceau SmartWater (my favorite; #1 recyclable, vapor distilled, and contains added calcium, magnesium, and potassium bicarbonate), 1-877-GLACEAU

Yogurt and Probiotics

Organic

365 Organic Fat Free Yogurt (various flavors), http://www.wholefoodsmarket.com

Stonyfield Organic 0% Fat (various flavors), http://www.Stonyfield.com

Stonyfield Oikos Organic Greek Yogurt (nonfat, various flavors), http://www.Stonyfield.com

Stonyfield Organic Super Smoothie (various flavors), http://www.Stonyfield.com

Nonorganic

Brown Cow All Natural 0% Fat Greek Yogurt (various flavors), http://www.BrownCowFarm.com

99% Fat Free Yoplait Yogurt, http://www.yoplait.com

Personal Care Products

Deodorant

Now Solutions Long-Lasting Deodorant Stick, Refreshing Lavender (paraben-free, no artificial colors or fragrances), http://www.nowfoods.com

Tom's of Maine Long Lasting Wild Lavender, http://www.tomsofmaine.com

Jason Calming Lavender Pure Natural Deodorant Stick (label states no aluminum, parabens, phthalates, or propylene glycol), http://www.jason-natural.com

Shampoo and Conditioner

Nature's Gate Shampoo/Conditioner (company also offers a complete line of personal care products), http://www.natures-gate.com

Skin Care

Epicuren After Bath Wake-Up Rosemary Moisturizer (and many other skin care products for all ages), http://www.epicuren.com

Vasseur Skincare (makes a variety of skin care products; my favorite for everyday use is Hand & Body Lotion; scent: winter mint, http://www.vasseurskin.com

Aveeno Baby Organic Harvest Lotion, http://www.aveeno.com

Aveeno Daily Moisturizing Lotion (fragrance free), http://www.aveeno.com

Toothpaste

Pure Propolis Toothpaste, http://www.holocuren.com

Nature's Gate natural toothpaste, http://www.natures-gate.com

12

Dr. Steve's Favorite Supplements for Moms and Dads

Although I believe in getting as many nutrients as possible from food by following a SuperFoods diet, I also believe that all men and women benefit from taking daily supplements. And since all children deserve to have two healthy parents, I'm providing lists of the supplements I would recommend for dads (and all men) as well as for moms (and women of all ages).

Always take your supplements with food, preferably a meal or a snack that contains all three macronutrients: protein, carbs, and fat. Take one or more of the following:

For Women during Prepregnancy, Pregnancy, and Lactation
Prenatal Pro, http://www.designsforhealth.com

For Women Nineteen Years and Older

Multi DFH Complete, http://www.designsforhealth.com

For Men Nineteen Years and Older (choose one)

The DOUBLEX Vitamin/Mineral/Phytonutrient difference, http://www.amway.com/shopnutrilite

Purity Products Perfect Multi, http://www.purityproducts.com

Med Op MaxiVision Whole Body Formula, http://www.medop.com

PhytoMulti—the Smart Multi, http://www.metagenics.com

For Men Only

Trunature Grape Seed and Resveratrol, distributed by Costco Wholesale Corporation, http://www.costco.com/diet-nutrition.html

Jarrow Alpha-Lipoic Acid with Biotin (take one a day with food), http://www.Jarrow.com

Omega-3 Supplements for Men and Women (choose one)

MaxiVision Omega-3 Formula, http://www.medop.com

OmegAvail with Vitamin D_3, K_1, and K_2, http://www.designsforhealth.com

Kirkland Signature Enteric Coated Omega-3 Fish Oil, http://www.costco.com

Nordic Naturals Ultimate Omega, http://www.nordicnaturals.com

Vital Choice Wild Alaskan Sockeye Salmon Oil, 1,000 mg, http://www.vitalchoice.com

Minerals for Men and Women Nineteen Years and Older

NatureMade Calcium, 750 mg, plus vitamins D and K, http://www.NatureMade.com

KAL Magnesium Glycinate 400, http://www.kalvitamins.com

Sun Harvest Amino Acid Chelated Magnesium, 250 mg, distributed by Amerifoods Trading Company; call 323-869-7500 to locate a store that sells Sun Harvest supplements

Vitamins/Phytonutrients/Antioxidants for Both Men and Women

Choline

Twin Lab Choline Caps, 300 mg, http://www.twinlab.com/product/choline-caps

Polyphenols

Proflavonol 90 or Proflavonol C, distributed by http://www.heatlhyvitamin.usana.com/

Truenature Cranberry, 300 mg, distributed by Costco Wholesale Corporation, http://www.costco.com/diet-nutrition.html

Sun Harvest Bilberry Extract, 100 mg, Vegetarian capsules, distributed by Amerifoods Trading Company; call 323-869-7500 to locate a store that sells Sun Harvest supplements (there is no website for this brand)

Co-Enzyme Q-10 (Co-Q-10)

Quinol Mega CoQ10 Ubiquinol, 100mg, active CoQ10, http://www.quinol.com

Vitamin C

Sun Harvest Bio C Caps, Vitamin C with Bioflavonoids, distributed by Amerifoods Trading Company; call 323-869-7500 to locate a store that sells Sun Harvest supplements

Vitamin D (choose one)

Nature Made D_3 1,000 IU (or 2,000 IU), http://www.NatureMade.com

Optimizers Vitamin D, 2,000 IU D_3 with vitamin K, 30 mcg (MK_4 and MK_7), http://healthyvitamin.usana.com/

Nordic Naturals Vitamin D_3 (in extra-virgin olive oil), 1,000 IU, http://www.nordicnaturals.com

Vital Choice D_3, 2,000 IU, in Wild Sockeye Salmon Oil, 300 mg, http://www.vitalchoice.com

Vitamin E (choose one)

Life Extenesion Gamma E Tocopherol with Sesame Lignans, http://www.LifeExtension.com

Life Extension Gamma E Tocopherol/Tocotrienols, http://www.LifeExtension.com

Kyani Sunset, a tocotrienol/salmon oil mix, http://www.kyani.net

Vitamin K

NOW Vitamin K_2, 100 mcg, http://www.nowfoods.com

Carlson Vitamin K_2, http://www.carlsonlabs.com

Superior Source Advanced Triple K (K1, K2[4], K2[7]) http://www.superiorsource1.com

L Carnitine

NOW Acetyl L Carnitine 500 mg, Vcaps, http://www.nowfoods.com

Spices

Cinnamon (pregnant women should check with their health-care providers before taking)

Puritan's Pride cinnamon (one or two 500 mg tablets daily), http://www.puritanspride.com

Curcumin

Gaia Turmeric Supreme, http://www.GaiaHerbs.com

Jarrow formula Turmeric Concentrate Curcumin 95, http://www.Jarrow.com

Natural Factors Turmeric & Bromelain 450 mg, http://www.naturalfactors.com/

Probiotics (choose one)

Bio-K+ Extra Strength Probiotic, http://www.biokplus.com

Sustenex Daily Probiotic, http://www.sustenex.com

Digestive Advantage, http://www.Schiffnutrition.com/

Theralac Probiotic Master Supplement 5 plus 2 Biotherapy (contains five probiotics and two prebiotics), http://www .master-supplements.com

Ultra Flora Plus DF Capsules, http://www.metagenics.com

Bibliography

Introduction

Barker DJ. Fetal origins of coronary heart disease. *British Medical Journal* 1995; 311: 171–174.

Barker DJ et al.Weight in infancy and death from ischemic heart disease. *Lancet* 1989; 2: 577–580.

Gluckman PD et al.Epigenetic mechanisms that underpin metabolic and cardiovascular diseases. *Nature Reviews Endocrinology* 2009; 5: 401–408.

Gluckman PD et al. Predictive adaptive responses and human evolution. *Trends in Ecology & Evolution* 2005; 20: 527–533.

Godfrey KM. Maternal regulation of fetal development and health in adult life. *European Journal of Obstetrics & Gynecology and Reproductive Biology* 1998; 78: 141–150.

Godfrey KM et al. Developmental origins of metabolic disease: Life course and intergenerational perspectives. *Trends in Endocrinology and Metabolism* 2010; 21: 199–205.

Hanson M et al. Developmental origins of noncommunicable disease: Population and public health implications. *American Journal of Clinical Nutrition* 2011; 94 (Suppl): 1754S–1758S.

Hanson MA et al. *Early life nutrition and lifelong health*. London: British Medical Association, 2009.

Jackson AA. Nutrient requirements to optimize neonatal growth. *American Journal of Clinical Nutrition* 2011; 94: 1394–1395.

Kaltiala-Heino R et al. Early puberty is associated with mental health problems in middle adolescence. *Social Science & Medicine* 2003; 57: 1055–1064.

Koletzko B. Early nutrition and its later consequences: New opportunities. *Advances in Experimental Medicine and Biology* 2005; 569: 1–12.

Koletzko B et al. The Early Nutrition Programming Project (EARNEST): 5 years of successful multidisciplinary collaborative research. *American Journal of Clinical Nutrition* 2011; 94 (Suppl): 1749S–1753S.

Lucas A. Programming by early nutrition in man. *Ciba Foundation Symposium* 1991; 156: 38–55.

Paul AM. *Origins: How the nine months before birth shape the rest of our lives.* New York: Free Press, 2010.

Pratt SG and Mathews K. *SuperFoods healthstyle: Simple changes to get the most out of life for the rest of your life.* New York: Harper, 2007.

Roseboom T et al. Effects of prenatal exposure to the Dutch famine on adult disease in later life: An overview. *Molecular and Cellular Endocrinology* 2001; 185: 93–98.

Sloboda DM et al. Age at menarche: Influences of prenatal and postnatal growth. *Journal of Clinical Endocrinology and Metabolism* 2007; 92: 46–50.

1. Fast-Track Your Fertility

Agarwal A et al. Clinical relevance of oxidative stress in male factor infertility: An update. *American Journal of Reproductive Immunology* 2008; 59 (1): 2–11.

Agarwal A et al. The effect of cell phone usage on semen analysis in men attending infertility clinic: An observational study. *Fertility and Sterility* 2008; 89 (1): 124–128.

Agarwal A et al. Role of antioxidants in treatment of male infertility: An overview of the literature. *Reproductive BioMedicine* 2004; 8: 616–627.

Anderson K et al. Lifestyle factors in people seeking infertility treatment: A review. *Australian and New Zealand Journal of Obstetrics and Gynecology* 2010; 50: 8–20.

Apples during pregnancy protect baby from asthma. Reuters. April 12, 2007. http://www.reuters.com/article/2007/04/12/us-apples-asthma-idUSCOL25916220070412.

Ashok A. Cell phones and male infertility: Dissecting the relationship. *Reproductive BioMedicine* 2007; 15 (3): 266–270.

Astaxanthin. Vitamins and Supplements, WebMD. http://www.webmd.com/vitamins-supplements/ingredientmono-1063-ASTAXANTHIN.aspx?activeIngredientId=1063&activeIngredientName=ASTAXANTHIN&source=1.

Ayaz FA et al. Phenolic acid contents of kale (*Brassica oleracea* L. var. *acephala* DC.) extracts and their antioxidant and antibacterial properties. *Food Chemistry* 2008; 107: 19–25.

Badman MK et al. The gut and energy balance: Visceral allies in the obesity war. *Science* 2005; 307: 1909–1914.

Beauchamp GK et al. Ibuprofen-like activity in extra-virgin olive oil. *Nature* 2005; 437: 45–46.

Berryman CE. Effects of almond consumption on the reduction of LDL-cholesterol: A discussion of potential mechanisms and future research directions. *Nutrition Reviews* 2011; 69 (4): 171–185.

Berthiller J et al. Smoking (active and passive) in relation to fertility, medically assisted procreation and pregnancy. *Journal of Gynecology, Obstetrics, and the Biology of Reproduction* 2005; SpecNo 1: 35: 47–54.

Bhatia J et al. Use of soy protein-based formulas in infant feeding. *Pediatrics* 2008; 121 (5): 1062–1068.

Bolûmar F et al. Caffeine intake and delayed conception: A European multicenter study on infertility and subfecundity. *American Journal of Epidemiology* 1997; 145: 324–334.

Boyer J et al. Apple phytochemicals and their health benefits. *Nutrition Journal* 2004; 3: 5.

Brugh III et al. Male factor infertility: Evaluation and management. *Medical Clinics of North America* 2004; 88: 367–385.

Buscemi S et al. Effects of red orange juice intake on endothelial function and inflammatory markers in adult subjects with increased cardiovascular risk. *American Journal of Clinical Nutrition* 2012; 95: 1089–1095.

Camargo A et al. Gene expression changes in mononuclear cells in patients with metabolic syndrome after acute intake of phenol-rich virgin olive oil. *BioMed Central Genomics* 2010; 11: 253.

Carlsen E et al. Evidence for decreasing quality of semen during the last 50 years. *British Medical Journal* 1992; 395: 609–613.

Cartea ME et al. Phenolic compounds in Brassica vegetables. *Molecules* 2011; 16: 251–280.

Cederroth CR et al. Potential detrimental effects of a phytoestrogen-rich diet on male fertility in mice. *Molecular and Cellular Endocrinology* 2010; 321 (2): 152–160.

Chen CY et al. Antioxidant capacity and bioavailability of oat avenanthramides. *Federation of American Societies for Experimental Biology Journal* 2005; 19: A1477.

Chen CY et al. Avenanthramides phenolic acids from oats are bioavailable and act synergistically with vitamin C to enhance hamster and human LDL resistance to oxidation. *Journal of Nutrition* 2004; 134 (6): 1459–1466.

Combaire FH et al. Combined conventional/antioxidant astaxanthin treatment for male infertility: A double-blind, randomized trial. *Asian Journal of Andrology* 2005; 7: 257–262.

Cornell study finds apples may reduce breast cancer risk. Orange Pippin. Accessed March 30, 2011. http://www.orangepippin.com/resources /health/apples-may-reduce-breast-cancer-risk.

Dawson E et al. Effect of ascorbic acid on male fertility. *Annals of the New York Academy of Sciences* 1987; 498: 312–323.

DeRuiter MC et al. Maternal transmission of risk for atherosclerosis. *Current Opinion in Lipidology* 2008; 19: 333–337.

Dillingham BL et al. Soy protein isolates of varied isoflavone content do not influence serum thyroid hormones in healthy young men. *Thyroid* 2007; 17 (2): 131–137.

Dreher ML. Pistachio nuts, composition and potential health benefits. *Nutrition Reviews* 2012; 70 (4): 234–240.

Enomoto T et al. Clinical effects of apple polyphenols on persistent allergic rhinitis: A randomized double-blind placebo-controlled parallel arm study. *Journal of Investigational Allergology and Clinical Immunology* 2006; 16 (5): 283–289.

Fardet A et al. New hypothesis for the health-protective mechanisms of whole-grain cereals: What is beyond fiber? *Nutrition Research Reviews* 2010; 23: 65–134.

Fresco P et al. The anticancer properties of dietary polyphenols and its relation with apoptosis. *Current Pharmaceutical Design* 2010; 16: 114–134.

Fuentes A et al. Recent cigarette smoking and assisted reproductive technologies outcome. *Fertility and Sterility* 2010; 93 (1): 89–95.

Garcia V et al. Dietary intake of flavonoids and asthma in adults. *European Respiratory Journal* 2005; 26 (3): 449–452.

Gatidis S et al. Phloridzin protects against erythrocyte cell membrane scrambling. *Journal of Agricultural and Food Chemistry* 2011; 59 (15): 8524–8530.

Ghanim H et al. Orange juice neutralizes the proinflammatory effects of a high-fat, high-carbohydrate meal and prevents endotoxin increase and toll-like receptor expression. *American Journal of Clinical Nutrition* 2010; 91: 940–949. Published erratum appears in *American Journal of Clinical Nutrition* 2011; 93: 674.

Gnoth C et al. Definition and prevalence of subfertility and infertility. *Human Reproduction* 2005; 20: 1144–1147.

Golomb BA et al. Association between more frequent chocolate consumption and lower body mass index. *Archives of Internal Medicine* 2012; 172 (6): 519–521.

Goyal A et al. The effects of dietary lycopene supplementation on human seminal plasma. *Journal of Compilation/British Journal of Urology International* 2007; 95: 1456–1460.

Grassi D et al. Cocoa reduces blood pressure and insulin resistance and improves endothelium-dependent vasodilation in hypertensives. *Hypertension* 2005; 46: 398–405.

Greb P. Blueberries and your health: Scientists study nutrition secrets of popular fruit. *Agricultural Research* May-June 2011: 9–16.

Greening D. Daily sex helps reduce sperm DNA damage and improve fertility. *Science Daily*, June 9, 2009, http://www.sciencedaily.com/releases/2009/06/09063007531.htm.

Gudmundsdottir SL. Hard training may decrease fertility in women. *Science Daily*, November 9, 2009, http://www.sciencedaily.com/releases2009/11/09111112057/htm.

Hartman J et al. Estrogen receptor beta in breast cancer—diagnostic and therapeutic implications. *Steroids* 2009; 74 (8): 635–641.

He RR et al. Protective effect of apple polyphenols against stress-provoked influenza viral infection in resistant mice. *Journal of Agricultural and Food Chemistry* 2011; 59 (8): 3730–3737.

Hlebowicz J et al. Effect of cinnamon on postprandial blood glucose, gastric emptying, and satiety in healthy subjects. *American Journal of Clinical Nutrition* 2007; 85 (6): 1552–1556.

Hooper L et al. Flavonoids, flavonoid-rich foods, and cardiovascular risk: A meta-analysis of randomized controlled trials. *American Journal of Clinical Nutrition* 2008; 88: 38–50.

Hudthagosol C et al. Pecans acutely increase plasma postprandial antioxidant capacity and catechins and decrease LDL oxidation in humans. *Journal of Nutrition* 2011; 141: 56–62.

Hunter DC et al. Consumption of gold kiwifruit reduces the severity and duration of selected upper respiratory tract infection symptoms and increases plasma vitamin C concentration in healthy older adults. *British Journal of Nutrition* 2011; 15: 1–11.

Irvine DS. Glutathione as a treatment for male infertility. *Reviews of Reproduction* 1996; 1: 6–12.

Jedrychowski W et al. Case-control study on beneficial effect of regular consumption of apples on colorectal cancer risk in a population with relatively low intake of fruits and vegetables. *European Journal of Cancer Prevention* 2010; 19 (1): 42–47.

Jung M et al. Influence of apple polyphenols on inflammatory gene expression. *Molecular Nutrition and Food Research* 2009; 53 (10): 1263–1280.

Jurenka JS. Therapeutic applications of pomegranate (Punica granatum L): A review. *Alternative Medicine Review* 2008; 13 (2): 128–144.

Kang NJ et al. Polyphenols as small molecular inhibitors of signaling cascades in carcinogenesis. *Pharmacology and Therapeutics* 2011; 130: 310–324.

Kao SH et al. Increase of oxidative stress in human sperm with lower motility. *Fertility and Sterility* 2008; 8: 1183–1190.

Katiyar SK. Green tea prevents non-melanoma skin cancer by enhancing DNA repair. *Archives of Biochemistry and Biophysics* 2011; 508 (2): 152–158.

Kelly SA et al. Whole-grain cereals for coronary heart disease (CHD). *Cochrane Database of Systematic Reviews* 2007; 2: CD00505.

Kidd P. Astaxanthin: Cell membrane nutrient with diverse clinical benefits and anti-aging potential. *Alternative Medicine Review* 2011; 16 (4): 355–364.

King DE et al. Effect of a high fiber diet vs. a fiber-supplemented diet on C-reactive protein level. *Archives of Internal Medicine* 2007; 167: 502–506.

Larsen SC et al. Magnesium intake and risk of type 2 diabetes: A meta-analysis. *Journal of Internal Medicine* 2007; 262: 208–214.

Lenzi A et al. Glutathione therapy for male infertility. *Archives of Andrology* 1992; 29: 65–68.

Lieke WJ et al. Salmon consumption by pregnant women reduces ex vivo umbilical cord endothelial cell activation. *American Journal of Clinical Nutrition* 2011; 94: 1418–1425.

Lim SS et al. The effect of obesity on polycystic ovary syndrome: A systematic review and meta-analysis. *Obesity Review* 2012; Oct 31.doi: 10.1111/j.1467-789×2102.01053.x. (Epub ahead of print)

Liu RH et al. Apples prevent mammary tumors in rats. *Journal of Agricultural and Food Chemistry* 2005; 53: 2341–2343.

Lopez-Miranda J et al. Olive oil and health: Summary of the international conference on olive oil and health consensus report. *Nutrition, Metabolism and Cardiovascular Diseases* 2010; 20: 284–294.

Ma J et al. Dual effects of phloretin and phloridzin on the glycation induced by methylglyoxal in model systems. *Chemical Research in Toxicology* 2011; 24 (8): 1304–1311.

Mann GE et al. Targeting the redox sensitive Nrf2-Keap1 defense pathway in cardiovascular disease: Protection afforded by dietary isoflavones. *Current Opinion in Pharmacology* 2009; 9 (2): 139–145.

Martinez-Gonzales MA et al. Nut consumption, weight gain and obesity: Epidemiological evidence. *Nutrition, Metabolism and Cardiovascular Diseases* 2010; 10: 1016.

Martinez-Tome M et al. Antioxidant properties of Mediterranean spice compared with common food additives. *Journal of Food Protection* 2001; 64: 1412–1419.

Mattes RD et al. Impact of peanuts and tree nuts on body-weight and healthy weight loss in adults. *Journal of Nutrition* 2008; 138: 174S-175S.

Meniola J et al. A low intake of antioxidant nutrients is associated with poor semen quality in patients attending fertility clinics. *Fertility and Sterility* 2010; 93 (4): 1128–1133.

Meydani M. Potential health benefits of avenanthramides of oats. *Nutrition Reviews* 2009; 67 (12): 731–735.

Miyazawa T et al. Plasma carotenoid concentrations before and after supplementation with astaxanthin in middle-aged and senior subjects. *Bioscience, Biotechnology, and Biochemistry* 2011; 75: 1856–1858.

Monagas M et al. Effect of cocoa powder on the modulation of inflammatory biomarkers in patients with high risk of cardiovascular disease. *American Journal of Clinical Nutrition* 2009; 90: 1144–1150.

Nagasako-Akazome Y et al. Apple polyphenols influence cholesterol metabolism in healthy subjects with relatively high body mass index. *Journal of Oleo Science* 2007; 58 (8): 417–428.

Nagasako-Akazome Y et al. Serum cholesterol-lowering effect of apple polyphenols in healthy subjects. *Journal of Oleo Science* 2005; 54 (3): 143–151.

National Institutes of Health, Office of Dietary Supplements. Dietary Supplement Fact Sheet: Zinc. http://ods.od.nih.gov/factsheets/Zinc-HealthProfessional/.

Nogueira L et al. Epicatechin enhances fatigue resistance and oxidative capacity in mouse muscle. *Journal of Physiology* 2011; 589 (18): 4615–4631.

Nothlings U et al. Intake of vegetables, legume, and fruit and risk for all-cause, cardiovascular and cancer mortality in a European diabetic population. *Journal of Nutrition* 2008; 138: 775–781.

Obikoya, G. The benefits of zinc. The Vitamins and Nutrition Center. http://www.vitamins-nutrition.org/vitamins/zinc.html.

Organic Facts. Health Benefits of Zinc. http://www.organicfacts.net/health-benefits/minerals/health-benefits-of-zinc.html.

Pan A et al. Red meat consumption and mortality. *Archives of Internal Medicine* 2012; 172 (7): 555–563.

Papanikolaou Y et al. Bean consumption is associated with greater nutrient intake, reduced systolic blood pressure, lower body weight and smaller waist circumference in adults: Results from the national health and nutrition examination survey, 1999–2002. *Journal of the American College of Nutrition* 2008; 27: 569–576.

Phillips KP et al. Human exposure to endocrine disruptors and semen quality. *Journal of Toxicology and Environmental Health* 2008; 11: 188–220.

Pipe EA et al. Soy protein reduces LDL cholesterol and the LDL cholesterol: HDL cholesterol and apolipoprotein B: apolipoprotein A-1 ratios in adults with type 2 diabetes. *Journal of Nutrition* 2009; 139 (9): 1700–1706.

Puel C et al. Prevention of bone loss by phloridzin, an apple polyphenol, in ovariectomized rats under inflammation conditions. *Calcified Tissue International* 2005; 77 (5): 311–318.

Rajaram S et al. Nuts, body weight and insulin resistance. *British Journal of Nutrition* 2006; 96: S79–S86.

Rasooly R et al. Inhibition of biological activity of staphylococcal enterotoxin A(SEA) by apple juice and apple polyphenols. *Journal of Agricultural and Food Chemistry* 2010; 58 (9): 5421–5426.

Rivlin RS. Historical perspective on the use of garlic. *Journal of Nutrition* 2001; 131 (3): 9515–9545.

Ruder EH. Diet and female fertility: Modifiable factors that may decrease time until pregnancy and increase fertility. *Clinical Nutrition Insight* 2009; 35 (2): 1–4.

Sandler B et al. Treatment of oligospermia with vitamin B-12. *Infertility* 1984; 7: 133–138.

Sarlos P et al. Comparative evaluation of the effect of antioxidants in the conservation of ram semen. *Acta Veterinaria Hungarica* 2002; 50: 235–245.

Scalbert A et al. Dietary polyphenols and the prevention of diseases. *Critical Reviews in Food Science and Nutrition* 2005; 45: 287–306.

Sermondade N et al. Obesity and Increased risk for oligoxoospermia and azoospermia. *Archives of Internal Medicine* 2012; 172 (5): 440–442.

Sesso HD et al. Tomato-based food products are related to clinically modest improvements in selected coronary biomarkers in women. *Journal of Nutrition* 2012; 142: 326–333.

Shen H et al. Detection of oxidative DNA damage in human sperm and its association with sperm function and male infertility. *Free Radical Biology and Medicine* 2000; 28: 529–536.

Shrime MG et al. Flavonoid-rich cocoa consumption affects multiple cardiovascular risk factors in a meta-analysis of short-term studies. *Journal of Nutrition* 2011; 141: 1982–1988.

Shu XO et al. Soy food intake and breast cancer survival. *Journal of the American Medical Association* 2009; 302 (22): 2437–2443.

Simopoulos AP and Cleland LG. Omega-6/omega-3 essential fatty acid ratio: The scientific evidence. *World Review of Nutrition and Dietetics* 2003; 92: 1–174.

Song Y et al. Soybean and soy isoflavone intake indicate a positive change in bone mineral density for 2 years in young Korean women. *Nutrition Research* 2008; 28 (1): 25–30.

Stangl V et al. The flavonoid phloretin suppresses stimulated expression of endothelial adhesion molecules and reduces activation of human platelets. *Journal of Nutrition* 2005; 135 (2): 172–178.

Stull AJ et al. Bioactives in blueberries improve insulin sensitivity in obese, insulin-resistant men and women. *Journal of Nutrition* 2010; 140: 1764–1768.

Swan S et al. The question of declining sperm density revisited: An analysis of 101 studies published 1934–1996. *Environmental Health Perspectives* 2000; 108: 961–966.

Torronen R et al. Berries modify the postprandial plasma glucose response to sucrose in healthy subjects. *British Journal of Nutrition* 2010; 103: 1094–1097.

Trinidad TP et al. The potential health benefits of legumes as a good source of dietary fibre. *British Journal of Nutrition* 2010; 103: 569–574.

Tvrda A et al. Impact of oxidative stress on male fertility—A review. *Acta Veterinaria Hungarica* 2011; 59 (4): 465–484.

Ursini F et al. Postprandial plasma lipid hydroperoxides: A possible link between diet and atherosclerosis. *Free Radical Biology and Medicine* 1998; 25: 250–252.

Van Bussel BCT et al. Fish consumption in healthy adults is associated with decreased circulating biomarkers of endothelial dysfunction and inflammation during a 6-year follow-up. *Journal of Nutrition* 2011; 141: 1719–1725.

Veeriah S et al. Intervention with cloudy apple juice results in altered biological activities of ileostomy samples collected from individual volunteers. *European Journal of Nutrition* 2008; 47 (5): 226–234.

Villegas R et al. Legume and soy food intake and the incidence of type 2 diabetes in the Shanghai Women's Health Study. *American Journal of Clinical Nutrition* 2008; 87: 162–167.

Vine MF, Tse CK, Hu P, Truong KY. Cigarette smoking and semen quality. *Fertility and Sterility* 1996; 65 (4): 835–842.

Vujkovic M et al. The preconception Mediterranean dietary pattern in couples undergoing in vitro fertilization / intracytoplasmic sperm injection treatment increases the chance of pregnancy. *Fertility and Sterility* 2010; 94: 2096–2101.

Wedick NM et al. Dietary flavonoid intakes and risk of type 2 diabetes in US men and women. *American Journal of Clinical Nutrition* 2012; 95: 925–933.

Westphal LM et al. Double-blind, placebo-controlled study of Fertility-Blend: A nutritional supplement for improving fertility in women. *Clinical and Experimental Obstetrics & Gynecology* 2006; 33 (4): 205–208.

Williams PG et al. Cereal grains, legumes, and weight management: A comprehensive review of the scientific evidence. *Nutrition Reviews* 2008; 66: 171–182.

Xu SZ et al. Multiple mechanisms of soy isoflavones against oxidative stress-induced endothelial injury. *Free Radical Biology and Medicine* 2009; 47 (2): 167–175.

Zessner H et al. Fractionation of polyphenol-enriched apple juice extracts to identify constituents with cancer chemopreventive potential. *Molecular Nutrition & Food Research* 2008; Suppl 1: S28–S44.

Zhang BM et al. Role of taurine supplementation to prevent exercise-induced oxidative stress in healthy young men. *Amino Acids* 2004; 26 (3): 267–271.

Zhang X et al. Carotenoid intakes and risk of breast cancer defined by estrogen receptor and progesterone receptor status: A pooled analysis of 18 prospective cohort studies. *American Journal of Clinical Nutrition* 2012; 95: 713–725.

Zhaoping L et al. Antioxidant-rich spice added to hamburger meat during cooking results in reduced meat, plasma, and urine malondialdehyde concentrations. *American Journal of Clinical Nutrition* 2010; 91: 1180–1184.

2. Baby-Proof Your Environment before You Conceive

American Lung Association. Air pollution: Metropolitan areas with the worst ozone pollution. *San Diego Union*, April 29, 2010, http://www.stateoftheair.org.

Boucher O et al. Prenatal exposure to polychlorinated biphenyls: A neuropsychologic analysis. *Environmental Health Perspectives* 2009; 117: 7–16.

Bruner-Tran KL et al. Dioxin-like PCBs and endometriosis. *Systems Biology in Reproductive Medicine* 2010; 56 (2): 132–146.

Canfield RL et al. Intellectual impairment in children with blood lead concentrations below 10 micrograms/dL. *New England Journal of Medicine* 2003; 348: 1517–1526.

Centers for Disease Control and Prevention (CDC). Third National Report on Human Exposure to Environmental Chemicals. Atlanta (GA), 2005. http://www.cdc.gov/exposurereport/.

Crinnion WJ. Chlorinated pesticides: Threats to health and importance of detection. *Alternative Medicine Review* 2009; 14 (4): 347–359.

Crinnion WJ. Maternal levels of xenobiotics that affect fetal development and childhood health. *Alternative Medicine Review* 2009; 14 (3): 212–222.

Environmental Defense Fund. PCBs in fish and shellfish. http://apps.edf.org/page.cfm?tagID=15904.

Goldschmidt L et al. Prenatal marijuana exposure and intelligence test performance at age 6. *Journal of the American Academy of Child and Adolescent Psychiatry* 2008; 47 (3): 254–263.

Gray KA et al. Prenatal marijuana use and child depression at age ten. *Neurotoxicology and Teratology* 1997; 19 (3): 245.

Hayes, WJ. *Pesticides studied in man*. Baltimore: Williams and Wilkins, 1982. Available at http://edis.ifas.ufl.edu/pi091.

Illinois Department of Public Health. Pyrethroid Insecticides. Environmental Health Fact Sheet. http://www.idph.state.il.us/envhealth/factsheets/pyrethroid.htm.

Lu C et al. Organic diets significantly lower children's dietary exposure to organophosphorous pesticides. *Environmental Health Perspectives* 2006; 114: 260–263.

Nour AM et al. Effect of maternal obesity and passive smoking on neonatal nucleated red blood cells. *International Journal of Food Safety, Nutrition and Public Health* 2010; 2 (1): 57–63.

Perera FP et al. A summary of recent findings on birth outcomes and developmental effects of prenatal ETS, PAH and pesticide exposures. *Neurotoxicology* 2005; 26 (4): 573–587.

Ranjit N et al. Bisphenol-A and disparities in birth outcomes: A review and directions for future research. *Journal of Perinatology* 2010; 30: 2–9.

Redmond E et al. Low-level prenatal exposure to organophosphate pesticides significantly lowers IQ in children. *Townsend Letter* 2012; 342: 58–62.

Rubin SR et al. Bisphenol A: Perinatal exposure and body weight. *Molecular and Cellular Endocrinology* 2009; 304 (1–2): 1–17.

U.S. Environmental Protection Agency. Pyrethroids and Pyrethrins. October 2012. http://www.epa.gov/oppsrrd1/reevaluation/pyrethroids-pyrethrins.html.

Van Goetz N et al. Bisphenol A: How the most relevant exposure sources contribute to total consumer exposure. *Risk Analysis* 2010; 30 (3): 473–487.

Wellenius GA et al. Ambient air pollution and the risk of acute ischemic stroke. *Archives of Internal Medicine* 2012; 172 (3): 229–234.

Weuve J et al. Exposure to particulate air pollution and cognitive decline in older women. *Archives of Internal Medicine* 2012; 172 (3): 219–227.

Winchester PD et al. Agrichemicals in surface water and birth defects in the United States. *Acta Paediatrica* 2009; 98: 664–669.

3. Prepare Your Body for Baby

Arora T et al. Fermentation potential of the gut microbiome: Implications for energy homeostasis and weight management. *Nutrition Reviews* 2011; 69 (2): 99–106.

Ayas NT et al. A prospective study of sleep duration and coronary heart disease in women. *Journal of the American Medical Association* 2003; 163: 205–209.

Bartz S et al. Pathogenesis and prevention of type 2 diabetes: Parental determinants, breastfeeding and early childhood nutrition. *Current Diabetes Reports* 2012; 12: 82–87.

Bezerra IN et al. Association between eating out of home and body weight. *Nutrition Reviews* 2012; 70 (2): 65–79.

Chan G. Pregnancy, in *Food and Nutrients in Disease Management*, edited by I Kohlstadt. New York: CRC Press, 2009, 669–684.

Dabelea D et al. Association of intrauterine exposure to maternal diabetes and obesity with type 2 diabetes in youth: The SEARCH case-control study. *Diabetes Care* 2008; 31: 1422–1426.

Denison FC et al. Increased maternal BMI is associated with an increased risk of minor complications during pregnancy with consequent cost implications. *BJOG: An International Journal of Obstetrics and Gynecology* 2009; 116: 1467–1472.

El-Toukhy T. *Being overweight doubles IVF miscarriage risk*. Paper presented at conference of European Society of Human Reproduction and Embryology, Rome, June 2010.

Fardini Y et al. Transmission of diverse oral bacteria to murine placenta: Evidence for the oral microbiome as a potential source of intrauterine infection. *Infection and Immunity* 2010; 78 (4): 1789–1796.

Fini L et al. Annurca apple polyphenols have potent demethylating activity and can reactivate silenced tumor suppressor genes in colorectal cancer cells. *Journal of Nutrition* 2007; 137: 2622–2628.

Gaskins AJ et al. Effect of daily fiber intake on reproductive function: The biocycle study. *American Journal of Clinical Nutrition* 2009; 90: 106–109.

Hamilton-Miller JM. Anti-cariogenic properties of tea (*Camellia sinensis*). *Journal of Medical Microbiology* 2001; 50: 299–302.

Hassam A et al. An α-linolenic acid-rich formula reduces oxidative stress and inflammation by regulating NF-$\kappa\beta$ in rats with TNBS-induced colitis. *Journal of Nutrition* 2010; 140: 1714–1721.

Hidde P et al. Sitting time and all-cause mortality risk in 222,497 Australian adults. *Archives of Internal Medicine* 2012; 172 (6): 494–500.

Huck O et al. Relationship between periodontal disease and preterm birth: Recent epidemiological and biological data. *Journal of Pregnancy* 2011. doi:10.1155/2011/164654.

Javaid MK et al. Maternal vitamin D status during pregnancy and childhood bone mass at age 9 years: A longitudinal study. *Lancet* 2006; 367 (9504): 36–43.

Kader YS et al. Periodontal disease and the risk of preterm birth and low birth weight: A meta-analysis. *Journal of Periodontology* 2005; 76 (2): 161–165.

Kalliomaki M et al. Early differences in fecal microbiota composition in children may predict overweight. *American Journal of Clinical Nutrition* 2008; 87: 534–538.

Kim OY et al. Independent inverse relationship between serum lycopene concentration and arterial stiffness. *Atherosclerosis* 2010; 208: 581–586.

Krakowiak P et al. Maternal metabolic conditions and risk for autism and other neurodevelopmental disorders. *Pediatrics* 2012; 129 (5): 1–8.

Krebs-Smith S et al. Americans do not meet federal dietary recommendations. *Journal of Nutrition* 2010; 140: 1832–1838.

Kujawska M et al. Cloudy apple juice protects against chemical-induced oxidative stress in rats. *European Journal of Nutrition* 2011; 50 (1): 53–60.

Kushiyama M et al. Relationship between intake of green tea and periodontal disease. *Journal of Periodontology* 2009; 80: 372–377.

Martin-Gronert M et al. Mechanisms linking suboptimal early nutrition and increased risk of type 2 diabetes and obesity. *Journal of Nutrition* 2010; 140: 662–666.

Meier-Evert HK et al. Effect of sleep loss on C-reactive protein, an inflammatory marker of cardiovascular risk. *Journal of the American College of Cardiology* 2004; 43: 678–683.

Mills JL et al. Maternal obesity and congenital heart defects: A population-based study. *American Journal of Clinical Nutrition* 2010; 91: 1543–1549.

Molloy AM et al. Maternal vitamin B12 status and risk of neural tube defects in a population with high neural tube defect prevalence and no folic acid fortification. *Pediatrics* 2009; 123: 917–923.

Morita K et al. Chlorophyll derived from chlorella inhibits dioxin absorption from the gastrointestinal tract and accelerates dioxin excretion in rats. *Environmental Health Perspectives* 2001; 109: 289–294.

National Institutes of Health, Office of Dietary Supplements. Dietary Supplement Fact Sheet: Vitamin B6. http://ods.od.nih.gov/factsheets/VitaminB6-QuickFacts/.

Nour AM et al. Effect of maternal obesity and passive smoking on neonatal nucleated red blood cells. *International Journal of Food Safety, Nutrition and Public Health* 2010; 3 (1): 57–63.

Offenbacher S et al. Effects of periodontal therapy on rate of preterm delivery: A randomized controlled study. *Obstetrics & Gynecology* 2009; 114 (3): 551–559.

Okah F. Weight rises for pregnant women and newborns. Paper presented at the annual meeting of the Pediatric Academic Societies, Vancouver, Canada, May 1–4, 2010.

Petermann A et al. GSTT1, a phase II gene induced by apple polyphenols, protects colon epithelial cells against genotoxic damage. *Molecular Nutrition & Food Research* 2009; 53 (10): 1245–1253.

Plagemann A et al. Long-term impact of neonatal breastfeeding on body weight and glucose tolerance in children of diabetic mothers. *Diabetes Care* 2002; 25: 16–22.

Ramagopalan SV et al. Expression of the multiple sclerosis-associated MHC Class II Allele *HLA-DRB1*1501* is regulated by vitamin D. *PLoS Genetics* 2009; 5 (2): e1000369.

Qi S et al. Adiposity and weight change in mid-life in relation to healthy survival after age 70 in women: Prospective cohort study. *British Medical Journal* 2009; 339: b3796.

Rasmussen S et al. Prepregnancy obesity and birth defects: What's next? *American Journal of Clinical Nutrition* 2010; 91: 1539–1540.

Roundtree R. Functional medicine approaches to detoxification. Paper presented at the annual conference Natural Supplements: An Evidence-Based Update, San Diego, January 19–22, 2012.

Salisberry PJ et al. Dynamics of early childhood overweight. *Pediatrics* 2005; 116: 1329–1338.

Stuebe AM et al. Maternal-recalled gestational weight gain, pre-pregnancy body mass index, and obesity in the daughter. *International Journal of Obesity* 2009; 33: 743–752.

Tinker SC et al. Folic acid intake among US women aged 15–44 years: National Health and Nutrition Examination Survey, 2003–2006. *American Journal of Preventive Medicine* 2010; 38: 534–542.

Whitaker KL et al. Comparing maternal and paternal intergenerational transmission of obesity risk in a large population-based sample. *American Journal of Clinical Nutrition* 2010; 91 (6): 1560–1567.

Wilson S MC et al. Oral contraceptive use: Impact on folate, vitamin B_6, and vitamin B_{12} status. *Nutrition Reviews* 2011; 69 (10): 572–583.

Yoo S et al. Antimicrobial traits of tea and cranberry-derived polyphenols against streptococcus mutans. *Caries Research* 2011; 45: 327–335.

You need iodine in pregnancy. Minnesota Birth. http://www.minnesotabirth
.com/pregnancy-and-birth/232-you-need-iodine-in-pregnancy.

Young BE et al. Maternal vitamin D status and calcium intake interact to affect
fetal skeletal growth in utero in pregnant adolescents. *American Journal
of Clinical Nutrition* 2012; 95: 1103–1112.

Zeisel SH et al. Is there a new component of the Mediterranean diet that reduces
inflammation? *American Journal of Clinical Nutrition* 2008; 87: 277–288.

5. The SuperFoods Way of Eating for Two

Allen S et al. Dietary supplementation with lactobacilli and bifidobacteria is
well tolerated and not associated with adverse events during late
pregnancy and early infancy. *Journal of Nutrition* 2010; 140: 483–488.

Artal A. Weight gain recommendations in pregnancy. *Expert Review of
Obstetrics & Gynecology* 2008; 3 (2): 143–145.

Bjorksten B. Environmental influences on the development of the immune
system: Consequences for disease outcome. *Nestlé Nutrition Workshop
Series: Pediatric Program* 2008; 61: 243–254.

Bondonno CP et al. Flavonoid-rich apples and nitrate-rich spinach augment
nitric oxide status and improve endothelial function in healthy men and
women: A randomized controlled trial. *Free Radical Biology and Medicine*
2012; 52: 95–102.

Bosscher D et al. Food-based strategies to modulate the composition of the
intestinal microbiota and their associated health effects. *Journal of
Physiology and Pharmacology* 2009; 60 (Suppl 6): 5–11.

Bruce KD et al. Maternal high-fat feeding primes steatohepatitis in adult mice
offspring, involving mitochondrial dysfunction and altered lipogenesis
gene expression. *Hepatology* 2009; 50: 1796–1808.

Bukowski R et al. Preconceptional folate supplementation and the risk of
spontaneous preterm birth: A cohort study. *Public Library of Science
Medicine* 2009; 6 (5): e1000061.

Cao H et al. Cinnamon extract and polyphenols affect the expression of
tristetraprolin, insulin receptor, and glucose transporter 4 in mouse 3T3-L1
adipocytes. *Archives of Biochemistry and Biophysics* 2007; 15 (2): 214–222.

Chan G. Pregnancy, in *Food and Nutrients in Disease Management*, edited by
I Kohlstadt. New York: CRC Press, 2009, 669–684.

Christian P et al. Maternal vitamin A and B-carotene supplementation and risk of bacterial vaginosis: A randomized controlled trial in rural Bangladesh. *American Journal of Clinical Nutrition* 2011; 94: 1643–1649.

Ciappio ED et al. Maternal one-carbon nutrient intake and cancer risk in offspring. *Nutrition Reviews* 2011; 69 (10): 561–571.

Crews D. Epigenetics, brain behavior, and the environment. *Hormones: International Journal of Endocrinology and Metabolism* 2010; 9 (1): 41–50.

Delespesse G. Is cleanliness to blame for increasing allergies? *Science Daily*, April 13, 2010.

Do R et al. The effect of chromosome 9p21 variants on cardiovascular disease may be predicted by dietary intake: Evidence from a case/control and prospective study. *Public Library of Science Medicine* 8 (10): e1001106. doi:10.1371.

Dole Nutrition Institute. *The Dole Nutrition Handbook*. Westlake Village, CA: Dole Food Company, 2010.

Donahue SMA et al. Prenatal fatty acid status and child adiposity at age 3 years: Results from a US pregnancy cohort. *American Journal of Clinical Nutrition* 2011; 93: 780–788.

Dugoua JJ et al. Probiotic safety in pregnancy: A systematic review and meta-analysis of randomized controlled trials of *Lactobacillus, Bifidobacterium*, and *Saccharomyces* spp. *Journal of Obstetrics and Gynaecology Canada* 2009; 31 (6): 542–552.

Fraser A et al. Association of maternal weight gain in pregnancy with offspring obesity and metabolic and vascular traits in childhood. *Circulation* 2010; 121: 2557–2564.

Friesen RW et al. Dietary arachidonic acid to EPA and DHA balance is increased among Canadian pregnant women with low fish intake. *Journal of Nutrition* 2009; 139: 2344–2350.

Goh YI et al. Prenatal multivitamin supplementation and rates of pediatric cancers: A meta-analysis. *Clinical Pharmacology & Therapeutics* 2007; 81: 685–691.

Hlebowicz J et al. Effects of 1 and 3 g cinnamon on gastric emptying, satiety, and postprandial blood glucose, insulin, glucose-dependent insulinotropic polypeptide, glucagon-like peptide 1, and ghrelin concentrations in healthy subjects. *American Journal of Clinical Nutrition* 2009; 89 (3): 815–821.

Hillier TA et al. Childhood obesity and metabolic imprinting: The ongoing effects of maternal hyperglycemia. *Diabetes Care* 2007; 30: 2287–2292.

Huang C et al. Early life exposure to the 1959–1961 Chinese famine has long-term health consequences. *Journal of Nutrition* 2010: 140; 1874–1878.

Jacobsen JL et al. Beneficial effects of polyunsaturated fatty acid on infant development: Evidence from the Inuit of arctic Quebec. *Journal of Pediatrics* 2008; 152: 356–364.

Jiang, R., et al. Nut and peanut butter consumption and risk of type 2 diabetes in women. *Journal of the American Medical Association* 2002; 288 (20): 2554–2560.

Kiel DW et al. Gestational weight gain and pregnancy outcomes in obese women: How much is enough? *Obstetrics & Gynecology* 2007; 110 (4): 752–758.

Kohlboeck G et al. Effect of fatty acid status in cord blood serum on children's behavioral difficulties at 10 years of age: Results from the LISAplus study. *American Journal of Clinical Nutrition* 2011; 94: 1592–1599.

Laitinen K et al. Dietary counseling and probiotic intervention initiated in early pregnancy modifies maternal adiposity over 12 months postpartum. *Obesity Facts* 2009; 2 (Suppl 2): 4.

Luoto R et al. Impact of maternal probiotic-supplemented dietary counseling on pregnancy outcome and prenatal and postnatal growth: A double-blind, placebo-controlled study. *British Journal of Nutrition* 2010; 103: 1792–1799.

Martin-Gronert M et al. Mechanisms linking suboptimal early nutrition and increased risk of type 2 diabetes and obesity. *Journal of Nutrition* 2010; 140: 662–666.

Mook-Kanamori DO et al. Risk factors and outcomes associated with first trimester fetal growth restriction. *Journal of the American Medical Association* 2010; 303 (6): 527–534.

Myhre R et al. Intake of probiotic food and risk of spontaneous preterm delivery. *American Journal of Clinical Nutrition* 2011; 93: 151–157.

Patelarou E et al. Association between biomarker-quantified antioxidant status during pregnancy and infancy and allergic disease during early childhood: A systematic review. *Nutrition Reviews* 2011; 69 (11): 627–664.

Perrin MC et al. Gestational diabetes as a risk factor for pancreatic cancer: A prospective cohort study. *BioMed Central Medicine* 2007; 5: 25.

Qin B et al. Cinnamon: Potential role in the prevention of insulin resistance, metabolic syndrome, and type 2 diabetes. *Journal of Diabetes Science and Technology* 2010 4 (3): 685–693.

Raqib R et al. Nutrition, immunology and genetics: Future perspectives. *Nutrition Reviews* 2009; 67 (Suppl. 2): S227–S236.

Rasmussen KM and Yaktine AL, eds. *Weight gain during pregnancy: Reexamining the guidelines.* Washington, DC: National Academies Press, 2009.

Schlotz A et al. Lower maternal folate status early in pregnancy is associated with childhood hyperactivity and peer problems in offspring. *Journal of Child Psychology and Psychiatry* 2010; 51 (5): 594–602.

Stuebe AM et al. Maternal recalled gestational weight gain, pre-pregnancy body mass index, and obesity in the daughter. *International Journal of Obesity* 2009; 33 (7): 743–752.

Toufektsian MC et al. Dietary flavonoids increase plasma very long-chain (n-3) fatty acids in rats. *Journal of Nutrition* 2011; 141: 37–41.

Tveden-Nyborg et al. Vitamin C deficiency in early postnatal life impairs spatial memory and reduces the number of hippocampal neurons in guinea pigs. *American Journal of Clinical Nutrition* 2009; 90: 540–546.

Tzounis X et al. Prebiotic evaluation of cocoa-derived flavonols in healthy humans by using a randomized, controlled, double-blind, crossover interventions study. *American Journal of Clinical Nutrition* 2011; 93: 62–72.

Vollset SE et al. Plasma total homocysteine, pregnancy complications, and adverse pregnancy outcomes: The Hordaland homocysteine study. *American Journal of Clinical Nutrition* 2000; 71 (4): 962–968.

Warner JO. Early life nutrition and allergy. *Early Human Development* 2007; 83: 777–783.

Wrotniak BH et al. Gestational weight gain and risk of overweight in the offspring at age 7 years in a multicenter, multiethnic cohort study. *American Journal of Clinical Nutrition* 2008; 87: 1818–1824.

Zeisel S et al. Choline: An essential nutrient for public health. *Nutrition Reviews* 2009; 67 (11): 615–623.

6. Optimize Your Lifestyle and Environment

Abel EL et al. Fetal alcohol syndrome is now leading cause of mental retardation. *Lancet* 1986; 2 (8517): 1222.

American College of Obstetricians and Gynecologists. Exercise during pregnancy and the postpartum period. *Obstetrics & Gynecology* 2002; 99: 171–173.

American Pregnancy Association. Need help putting down that cigarette? May 2011. http://www.americanpregnancy.org/pregnancyhealth/smoking.html.

Ayas NT et al. A prospective study of sleep duration and coronary heart disease in women. *Journal of the American Medical Association* 2003; 163: 205–209.

Ayyanan A et al. Perinatal exposure to bisphenol A increases adult mammary gland progesterone response and cell number. *Molecular Endocrinology* 2011; 25 (11): 1915–1923.

Banks S et al. Behavioral and physiological consequences of sleep restriction. *Journal of Clinical Sleep Medicine* 2007; 3 (5): 519–528.

Bassetti GI et al. Sleep and stroke. *Seminars in Neurology* 2005; 25 (1): 19–32.

Boyles S. Pregnant women don't get enough exercise. WebMD, April 1, 2010. http://www.webmd.com/baby/news/20100402/pregnant-women-dont-get-enough-exercise.

Braun JM et al. Impact of early-life bisphenol A exposure on behavior and executive function in children. *Pediatrics* 2011; 128 (5): 873–882.

Bruce CR et al. Muscle oxidative capacity is a better predictor of insulin sensitivity than lipid status. *Journal of Clinical Endocrinology and Metabolism* 2003; 88 (11): 5441–5451.

Chan G. Pregnancy, in *Food and Nutrients in Disease Management*, edited by I Kohlstadt. New York: CRC Press, 2009, 669–684.

Cordain L. *The Paleo Diet*. Hoboken, NJ: John Wiley & Sons, 2001.

Damgaard IN et al. Persistent pesticides in human breast milk and cryptorchidism. *Environmental Health Perspectives* 2006; 114 (7): 1133–1138.

Definition of folic acid. Medicine Net. http://www.medterms.com/script/main/art.asp?articlekey=11365.

Dolinoy DC et al. Maternal nutrient supplementation counteracts bisphenol A-induced DNA hypomethylation in early development. *Proceedings of the National Academy of Science USA* 2007; 104: 13035–13061.

Durmaz E et al. Plasma phthalate levels in pubertal gynecomastia. *Pediatrics* 2010; 125 (1): 122–129.

Engel S et al. Prenatal phthalate exposure is associated with childhood behavior and executive functioning. *Environmental Health Perspectives* 2010; 118: 565–571.

Epel E et al. Stress may add bite to appetite in women: A laboratory study of stress-induced cortisol and eating behavior. *Psychoneuroendocrinology* 2001; 26 (1): 37–49.

Evenson KR et al. National trends in self-reported physical activity and sedentary behaviors among pregnant women: NHANES, 1999–2006. *Preventive Medicine* 2010; 50 (3): 123–128.

Exercise and depression. WebMD. http://www.webmd.com/depression/guide/exercise-depression.

Exposure to phthalates may be a risk factor for low-birth weight in infants. *Science Daily*, June 25, 2009. http://www.sciencedaily.com/releases/2009/06/090625074408.htm.

Foltran F et al. Effect of alcohol consumption in prenatal life, childhood, and adolescence on child development. *Nutrition Reviews* 2011; 69 (11): 642–659.

Forcelli PA et al. Teratogenic effects of maternal antidepressant exposure on neural substrates of drug-seeking behavior in offspring. *Addiction Biology* 2008; 13: 52–62.

Frederick AL et al. Drugs, biogenic amine targets and the developing brain. *Developmental Neuroscience* 2009; 31 (2): 7–22.

Gilden RC et al. Pesticides and health risks. *Journal of Obstetric, Gynecologic, and Neonatal Nursing* 2010; 39: 103–110.

Gutierrez J et al. Slimming slumber? How sleep deprivation manipulates appetite and weight. *Nutrition Today* 2010; 45 (2): 77–81.

Hall KD et al. Quantification of the effect of energy imbalance on bodyweight. *Lancet* 2011; 378: 826–837.

Hernandez-Alvarez MI et al. Subjects with early-onset type 2 diabetes show defective activation of the skeletal muscle PGC-1α/mitofusin-2 regulatory pathway in response to physical activity. *Diabetes Care* 2010; 33 (3): 645–651.

Hublin C et al. Sleep and mortality: A population-based 22 year follow-up study. *Sleep* 2007; 30 (10): 1245–1253.

Kaiser Permanente, Division of Research. In utero exposure to BPA may adversely affect male genital development. August 29, 2011. http://www.dor.kaiser.org/external/DORExternal/news/press_releases/press_release.aspx?id=8208&terms=BPA.

Kim BN et al. Phthalates exposure and attention-deficit/hyperactivity disorder in school-age children. *Biological Psychiatry* 2009; 16(10): 958–963.

Kopp L et al. Direct and passive prenatal nicotine exposure and the development of externalizing psychopathology. *Child Psychiatry and Human Development* 2007; 38: 255–269.

Lovasi GS et al. Chlorpyrifos exposure and urban residential environment characteristics as determinants of early childhood neurodevelopment. *American Journal of Public Health* 2011; 101 (1): 63–70.

Lunder S. Tips to avoid BPA exposure. Environmental Working Group. October 2008. http://www.ewg.org/bpa/tipstoavoidbpa.

March of Dimes. Alcohol during pregnancy. http://www.marchofdimes.com /pregnancy/alcohol_indepth.html.

March of Dimes. Smoking during pregnancy. http://www.marchofdimes.com /pregnancy/alcohol_smoking.html?gclid=CNz1tI3q9a0CFUFN4AodXxC7rQ.

Meier-Ewert HK et al. Effect of sleep loss on C-reactive protein, an inflammatory marker of cardiovascular risk. *Journal of the American College of Cardiology* 2004; 43: 678–883.

The Michigan Maternal Infant Cohort Study (Fein et al. 1984; Jacobson et al. 1985, 1990a, b).

Nedeltcheva AV et al. Sleep curtailment is accompanied by increased intake of calories from snacks. *American Journal of Clinical Nutrition* 2009; 89: 126–133.

Pedersen LH et al. Selective serotonin reuptake inhibitors in pregnancy and congenital malformations: Population-based cohort study. *British Medical Journal* 2009; 339: b3569.

Perzanowski MS et al. Prenatal acetaminophen exposure and risk of wheeze at age 5 years in an urban low-income cohort. *Thorax* 2010; 65 (2): 118–123.

Poudevigne MS, O'Connor PJ. Physical activity and mood during pregnancy. *Medicine and Science in Sports and Exercise* 2005; 37 (8): 1374–1380.

Pratt S. *SuperHealth: 6 simple steps, 6 easy weeks, 1 longer healthier life*. New York: Dutton, 2009.

Rochman B. Smoking during pregnancy may result in uncoordinated kids. *Time*, September 28, 2010.

Sharpe RM. Environmental and lifestyle effects on spermatogenesis. *Philosophical Transactions of the Royal Society B: Biological Sciences* 2010; 365: 1697–1712.

Skakkeback NE et al. Testicular dysgenesis syndrome: An increasingly common developmental disorder with environmental aspects: Opinion. *Human Reproduction* 2001; 16(5): 972–978.

St-Onge MP et al. Sleep restriction leads to increased activation of brain regions sensitive to food stimuli. *American Journal of Clinical Nutrition* 2012; 95: 818–824.

Swan SH et al. Decrease in anogenital distance among male infants with prenatal phthalate exposure. *Environmental Health Perspectives* 2005; 8 (113): 1056–1061.

U.S. Department of Health and Human Services. *2008 physical activity guidelines for Americans: Be active, healthy, and happy!* http://www.health.gov/paguidelines.

U.S. Environmental Protection Agency. Health effects of PCBs. http://www.epa.gov/epawaste/hazard/tsd/pcbs/pubs/effects.htm.

U.S. Environmental Protection Agency. Summary of the Toxic Substances Control Act. 1976. http://www.epa.gov/lawsregs/laws/tsca.html.

Van Couter E et al. Impact of sleep and sleep loss on neuroendocrine and metabolic function. *Hormone Research* 2007; 67 (Suppl): 2–9.

Van Gelder MHJ et al. Teratogenic mechanism of medical drugs. *Human Reproduction Update* 2010; 16 (4): 378–394.

Van Gotz N et al. Bisphenol A: How the most relevant exposure sources contribute to total consumer exposure. *Consumer Analysis* 2010; 30: 473–487.

Wen SW et al. Maternal exposure to folic acid antagonists and placenta-mediated adverse pregnancy outcomes. *Canadian Medical Association Journal* 2008; 179 (12): 1263–1268.

Wisconsin Department of Health Services. Polychlorinated Biphenyls (PCBs) and Your Health. Fact Sheet. http://www.dhs.wisconsin.gov/eh/hlthhaz/fs/pcblink.htm.

Wohlfahrt-Veje C. et al. Testicular dysgenesis syndrome: Foetal origin of adult reproductive problems. *Clinical Endocrinology* 2000; 71: 459–465.

Woodruff TJ et al. Environmental chemicals in pregnant women in the United States: NHANES, 2003–2004. *Environmental Health Perspectives* 2011; 119: 878–885.

Woods SC et al. Adiposity signals and the control of energy homeostasis. *Nutrition* 2000; 16: 894–902.

Yonkers KA et al. The management of depression during pregnancy: A report from the American Psychiatric Association and the American College of Obstetricians and Gynecologists. *General Hospital Psychiatry* 2009; 31: 403–413.

Zhang Y et al. Phthalate levels and low birth weight: A nested case-control study of Chinese newborns. *Journal of Pediatrics* 2009; 155: 500–504.

8. Breast-Feeding Your Baby

Alves JGB et al. Breastfeeding protects against type I diabetes mellitus: A case-sibling study. *Breastfeeding Medicine* 2012; 7 (1): 25–28.

American Academy of Pediatrics. *Public statement on breastfeeding and the use of human milk.* 2012 http://pediatrics.aappublications.org/content/early/2012/02/peds.2011–3552.

Barennes H et al. Breast-milk substitutes: A new-old threat for breastfeeding policy in developing countries: A case study in a traditionally high breastfeeding country. *Public Library of Science* 2012; 7(2): e30634.

Beard J. Iron deficiency alters brain development and functioning. *Journal of Nutrition* 2003; 133: 1468S–1472S.

Belderbos ME et al. Breastfeeding modulates neonatal innate immune responses: A prospective birth cohort study. *Pediatric Allergy and Immunology* 2011; 23: 65–74.

Bode L. Human milk oligosaccharides: Prebiotics and beyond. *Nutrition Reviews* 2009; 67 (Suppl. 2): 5183–5191.

Boerner BP et al. Type I diabetes: Role of intestinal microbiome in humans and mice. *Annals of the New York Academy of Science* 2011; 1243: 103–118.

Centers for Disease Control. *Breastfeeding national immunization survey data,* 2007, http://www.edc.gov/breastfeeding/data/NIS_data/.

Corvalan C et al. Effect of growth on cardiometabolic status at 4 years of age. *American Journal of Clinical Nutrition* 2009; 90: 547–555.

Cunningham-Rundles S et al. Role of nutrients in the development of neonatal immune response. *Nutrition Reviews* 2009; 67 (Suppl. 2): 5152–5163.

Deshmukh-Taskar P et al. Tracking of overweight status from childhood to young adulthood: The Bogalusa heart study. *European Journal of Clinical Nutrition* 2006; 60 (1): 48–57.

Fernandes TA et al. Prepregnancy weight, weight gain during pregnancy, and exclusive breastfeeding in the first month of life in Rio de Janeiro, Brazil. *Journal of Lactation* 2012; 28 (1): 55–61.

The function of iron supplements. http://www.pharmics.com/resources/iron/.

Gale C et al. Effect of breastfeeding compared with formula feeding on infant body composition: A systematic review and meta-analysis. *American Journal of Clinical Nutrition* 2012; 95: 656–669.

Garcia MV et al. The influence of the type of breastfeeding on middle ear conditions in infants. *Brazilian Journal of Otorhinolaryngology* 2012; 78 (1): 8–14.

Gunderson P et al. Duration of lactation and incidence of the metabolic syndrome in women of reproductive age according to gestational diabetes mellitus status: A 20-year prospective study in coronary artery risk development in young adults. *Diabetes* 2010; 59: 495–504.

Harder T et al. Duration of breastfeeding and risk of overweight: A meta-analysis. *American Journal of Epidemiology* 2005; 162 (5): 397–403.

Hoppu U et al. Vitamin C in breast milk may reduce the risk of atopy in the infant. *Free Radical Research* 2006; 40 (2): 199–206.

Huff L et al. Body image concerns and reduced breastfeeding duration in primiparous overweight and obese females. *American Journal of Human Biology* 2012; 24: 339–349.

Jackson JG et al. Major carotenoids in mature human milk: Longitudinal and diurnal patterns. *Nutritional Biochemistry* 1998; 9: 2–9.

Jansson L et al. Vitamin E and fatty acid composition of human milk. *American Journal of Clinical Nutrition* 1981; 34: 8–13.

Jantscher-Krenn E et al. Human milk oligosaccharides and their potential benefits for the breast-fed neonate. *Minerva Pediatrica* 2012; 64: 83–99.

Jedrychowski W et al. Effect of exclusive breastfeeding on the development of children's cognitive function in the Krakow prospective birth cohort study. *European Journal of Pediatrics* 2012; 171 (1): 151–158.

Khachik F et al. Identification, quantification and relative concentrations of carotenoids and their metabolites in human milk and serum. *Analytical Chemistry* 1997; 69: 1873–1881.

Khan NC et al. The contribution of plant foods to the vitamin A supply of lactating women in Vietnam: A randomized controlled trial. *American Journal of Clinical Nutrition* 2007; 85: 1112–1120.

Koletzko B. et al. Lower protein in infant formula is associated with lower weight up to age 2 years: A randomized clinical trial. *American Journal of Clinical Nutrition* 2009; 89 (6): 1836–1845.

Labayen I et al. Exclusive breastfeeding duration and cardiorespiratory fitness in children and adolescents. *American Journal of Clinical Nutrition* 2012; 95: 498–505.

Larson-Meyer DE et al. Ghrelin and peptide YY postpartum in lactating and nonlactating women. *American Journal of Clinical Nutrition* 2010; 91: 366–372.

Ley SH et al. Associations of prenatal metabolic abnormalities with insulin and adiponectin concentrations in human milk. *American Journal of Clinical Nutrition* 2012; 95: 867–874.

Martin JA et al. Births: Final data for 2007. *National Vital Statistics Reports* 2010; 58: 1–85.

Martin RM et al. Breastfeeding and atherosclerosis intima-media thickness and plaques at 65-year follow-up of the Boyd Orr cohort. *Arteriosclerosis, Thrombosis, and Vascular Biology* 2005; 25: 1482–1488.

Martin V et al. Sharing of bacteria strains between breast milk and infant feces. *Journal of Human Lactation* 2012; 28 (1): 36–44.

Metzger AM et al. Human milk versus formula feeding among preterm infants: Short-term outcomes. *American Journal of Perinatology* 2012; 29: 121–126.

Min BR et al. Comparative antimicrobial activity of tannin extracts from perennial plants on mastitis pathogens. *Scientific Research and Essay* 2008; 3 (2): 66–73.

Morrison JA et al. Childhood predictors of adult type 2 diabetes at 9- and 26-year follow-ups. *Archives of Pediatrics and Adolescent Medicine* 2010; 164 (1): 53–60.

Owen CG et al. Effect of infant feeding on the risk of obesity across the life course: A quantitative review of published evidence. *Pediatrics* 2005; 115 (5): 1367–1377.

Pisacane A et al. Breastfeeding and risk for fever after immunization. *Pediatrics* 2010; 125: e1448–e1452.

Prior E et al. Breastfeeding after cesarean section delivery: A systematic review and meta-analysis of world literature. *American Journal of Clinical Nutrition* 2012; 95: 1113–1135.

Riskin A et al. Changes in immunomodulatory constituents of human milk in response to active infection in the nursing infant. *Pediatric Research* 2012; 71 (2): 220–225.

Scalbert A et al. Polyphenols: Antioxidants and beyond. *American Journal of Clinical Nutrition* 2005; 81 (1): 215S–217S.

Schack-Nielsen L et al. Late introduction of complementary feeding, rather than duration of breastfeeding, may protect against adult overweight. *American Journal of Clinical Nutrition* 2010; 91: 619–627.

Scott JA et al. The relationship between breastfeeding and weight status in a national sample of Australian children and adolescents. *BioMed Central Public Health* 2012; 12: 107.

Serpero LD et al. Human milk and formulae: Neurotrophic and new biological factors. *Early Human Development* 2012; 88: S9–S12.

Sonnenschein–van der Voort AMM. et al. Duration and exclusiveness of breastfeeding and childhood asthma-related symptoms. *European Respiratory Journal* 2012; 39: 81–89.

Soto-Ramirez N et al. Breastfeeding is associated with increased lung function at 18 years of age: A cohort study. *European Respiratory Journal* 2012; 39: 985–991.

Stuebe AM et al. Lactation and incidence of premenopausal breast cancer. *Archives of Internal Medicine* 2009; 169 (15): 1364–1371.

Tveden-Nyborg P et al. Vitamin C deficiency in early postnatal life impairs spatial memory and reduces the number of hippocampal neurons in guinea pigs. *American Journal of Clinical Nutrition* 2009; 90: 540–546.

UNICEF. *Infant and young child feeding*, 2008, http//www.unicef.org/nutrition/index.breastfeeding.htmi.

Villalpando S et al. Early and late effects of breast-feeding: Does breast-feeding really matter? *Biology of the Neonate* 1998; 74: 177–191.

Wiedmeier JE et al. Early postnatal nutrition and programming of the preterm neonate. *Nutrition Reviews* 2011; 69 (2): 76–82.

Woo JG et al. Human milk adiponectin affects infant weight trajectory during the second year of life. *Journal of Pediatric Gastroenterology and Nutrition* 2012; 54: 532–539.

9. Sleep, Stress, and Physical Activity

Abou-Dakn M et al. Psychological stress and breast disease during lactation. *Breastfeeding Review* 2009; 17 (3): 19–26.

Adegboye A et al. Diet or exercise, or both, for weight reduction in women after childbirth. *Cochrane Collaboration* 2008; 4: 1–40.

Association of Women's Health, Obstetric and Neonatal Nurses. Sleep quality in women with and without postpartum depression. *Journal of Obstetric, Gynecologic, & Neonatal Nursing* 2008; 37 (6); 722–737.

Blyton DM et al. Lactation is associated with an increase in slow-wave sleep in women. *Journal of Sleep Research* 2002; 11(4): 297–303.

Breastfeeding: Soothes baby and mom. *Science Daily,* August 5, 2005. http://www.sciencedaily.com/releases/2005/08/050805175820.htm.

Cleveland Clinic. Diet, exercise, stress, and the immune system. http://my.clevelandclinic.org/disorders/chronic_fatigue_syndrome/hic_diet_exercise_stress_and_the_immune_system.aspx.

Dorheim SK et al. Sleep and depression in postpartum women: A population-based study. *Sleep* 2009; 32 (7): 847–855.

Engler AC et al. Breastfeeding may improve nocturnal sleep and reduce infantile colic: Potential role of breast milk melatonin. *European Journal of Pediatrics* 2012; 171: 729–732.

Evenson KR et al. Physical activity beliefs, barriers, and enablers among postpartum women. *Journal of Women's Health* 2009; 18 (12): 1925–1934.

Fleshner, F. Physical activity and stress resistance: Sympathetic nervous system adaptations prevent stress-induced immunosuppression. *Exercise & Sport Sciences Reviews* 2005; 33 (3): 120–126.

Gunderson EP et al. Association of fewer hours of sleep at 6 months postpartum with substantial weight retention at 1 year postpartum. *American Journal of Epidemiology* 2008; 167: 178–187.

Gutierrez J et al. Slimming slumber? How sleep deprivation manipulates appetite and weight. *Nutrition Today* 2010; 45 (2): 77–81.

Keith DR et al. The effect of music-based listening interventions on the volume, fat content, and caloric content of breast-milk produced by mothers of premature and critically ill infants. *Advances in Neonatal Care* 2012; 12 (2): 112–119.

Laugero KD. Obesity, the economic meltdown, and the gut feeling for the foods we choose to eat. *Clinical Nutrition Insight* 2010; 36 (5): 1–4.

Mayo Clinic. Exercise and stress: Get moving to manage stress. http://www.mayoclinic.com/health/exercise-and-stress/SR00036.

Mayo Clinic. Walking: Trim your waistline, improve your health. http://www.mayoclinic.com/health/walking/HQ01612.

Montgomery-Downs HE et al. Infant feeding methods and maternal sleep and daytime functioning. *Pediatrics* 2010; 126: e1562–e1568.

Nedeltcheva AV et al. Insufficient sleep undermines dietary efforts to reduce adiposity. *Annals of Internal Medicine* 2010; 153: 435–441.

Park BJ et al. The physiological effects of *shinrin-yoku* (taking in the forest atmosphere or forest bathing): Evidence from field experiments in 24 forests across Japan. *Environmental Health Preventive Medicine* 2010; 15: 18–26.

Sanchez CL et al. The possible role of human milk nucleotides as sleep inducers. *Nutritional Neuroscience* 2009; 12 (1): 2–8.

Taveras EM et al. Association of maternal short sleep duration with adiposity and cardiometabolic status at 3 years postpartum. *Obesity* 2011; 19: 171–178.

Tong J et al. Ghrelin suppresses glucose-stimulated insulin secretion and deteriorates glucose tolerance in healthy humans. *Diabetes* 2010; 59 (9): 2145–2151.

U.S. Department of Health and Human Services. Physical activity guidelines for Americans, chapter 7: Additional considerations for some adults. http://www.health.gov/paguidelines/guidelines/chapter7.aspx.

Index